With Tea

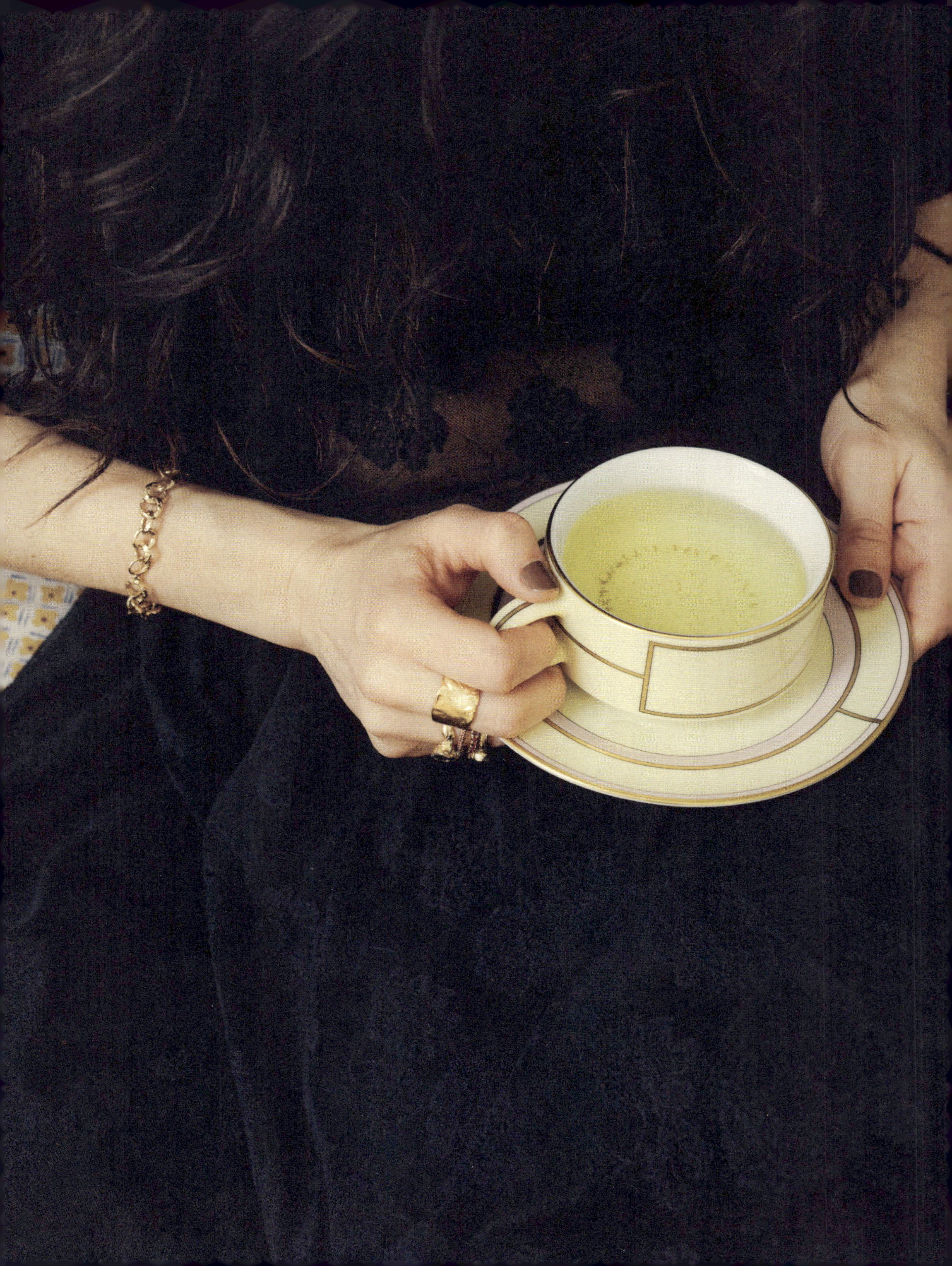

With Tea

Culture, Accoutrements, and Rituals

Maria Geyman

RIZZOLI
NEW YORK
New York · Paris · London · Milan

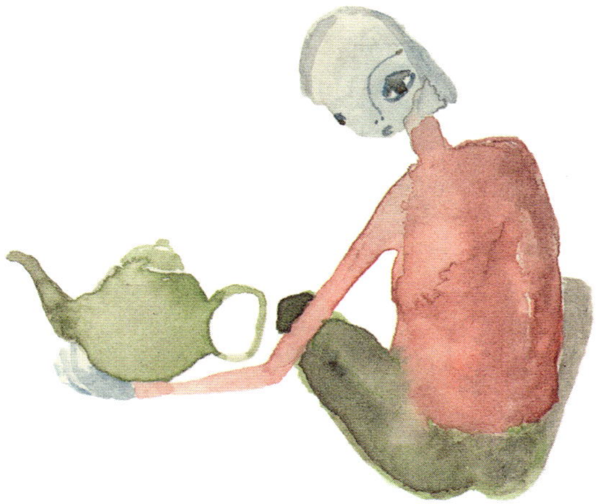

Contents

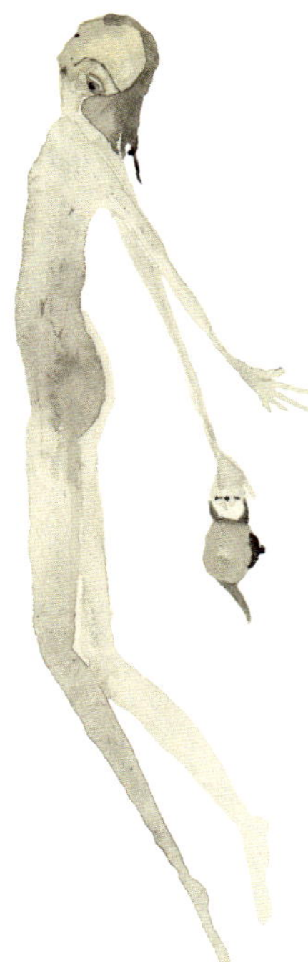

To my daughter, Mona Rita Seftel,
and my grandmother, Rita Zenovievna Geyman

Introduction

I like to make tea for friends and strangers alike, and I love when people make tea for me. When I consider my early experiences with tea culture, I think of drinking pots of black tea as a child while playing cards on the porch during summers with my grandparents in upstate New York. I think of having chai on the train in India, looking out at rolling tea farms alongside rice fields in Japan, and watching any French New Wave film and admiring the casually laid out tea sets. My perspective on tea culture comes as a New Yorker from the Soviet diaspora, as a board-certified naturopathic doctor, as someone who has written about tea for fashion magazines, and as a host who has spent years throwing tea parties.

I grew up drinking Indian black tea with my Ukrainian-Jewish family, and later moved to Portland, Oregon, to go to graduate school to earn my doctorate, where I spent years studying medicinal herbs. In place of black tea, I made teas from these (new-to-me) herbs in my family's beautiful Soviet-era teaware. Using these family heirlooms in new ways excited me, and I saw a connection between a very specific cultural practice that my immigrant parents brought to the United States—drinking black tea—and that of a very modern culture of herbalism. Modern not in the sense that the ideas are new—herbalism is ancient—but there is an undeniably growing popularity in herbalism, nutrition, and wellness. Tea culture became a way for me to weave my heritage into the new places I was seeing and the ideas I was discovering as a young person.

In my twenties, I traveled a lot and began to recognize tea as an international symbol of hospitality. My travels, my education, and my family story initially inspired me to begin my tea company, Masha Tea. Its existence has enabled me to travel to more tea farms and hubs of tea culture, to dig deeper into my ancestry, and to become interested in discussing contemporary tea culture, and therefore the tea culture of the future.

For Masha Tea, I focus on teas and herbs grown in the U.S., Japan, India, and the Mediterranean, simply because those are the places where I've visited and source tea. Tea culture is vast—crossing continents—so if I've left out regions it is not due to purposeful omission, but rather because

I wanted to focus on what I know best and have experienced firsthand. Tea seems to infiltrate cultures, and because we so often see it served in dusty little bags, we forget that tea is a plant, it grows somewhere, it is agriculture. Some places and people grow tea with more care than others. How tea is farmed, processed, stored, packaged, and sold all impact the tea in our cups.

Tea is so much more than a beverage—it is a lifestyle. An evergreen, the tea plant, *Camellia sinensis*, has been cultivated for thousands of years and is the source of the most widely consumed beverage in the world after water. Tea drinking has crossed cultures, and it has started wars and love stories alike.

How curious, the global interest in tea. It's not food, it doesn't give us sustenance. Maybe its allure comes from that elusive sense of calm and ease that we so desperately want as humans. We consider the fact that everything moves too fast, our cortisol levels are high, there is so much to worry about as a modern problem. But maybe more than a modern problem, it's a human problem. And one of the places that we turn to in order to alleviate our worries is a cup of tea.

I'm convinced there's a tea for every life event. Think about the mundane—mornings and Mondays—and the extraordinary—falling in love or losing someone you love. How you feel in those moments can be complemented by different teas. I write "complemented" rather than "enhanced, or muted, or healed" because it's truer. Tea acts subtly, accompanying those moments of reflection while you experience the waves of everyday life.

Tea has existed for thousands of years and tea drinking has stood the test of time. In this book, I'll describe the myths and legends behind tea origins; consider the implications of colonialism on modern tea culture; discuss tea accoutrements; help you to entertain with style and ease, and create your own tea rituals; and share ways to use teas and herbs medicinally. You will certainly learn how to make a great cup of tea, but more than that, I hope you'll expand your view of what tea culture is, learn how tea can enhance your well-being, and experiment with crafting a calmer, chicer, and more peaceful life with tea.

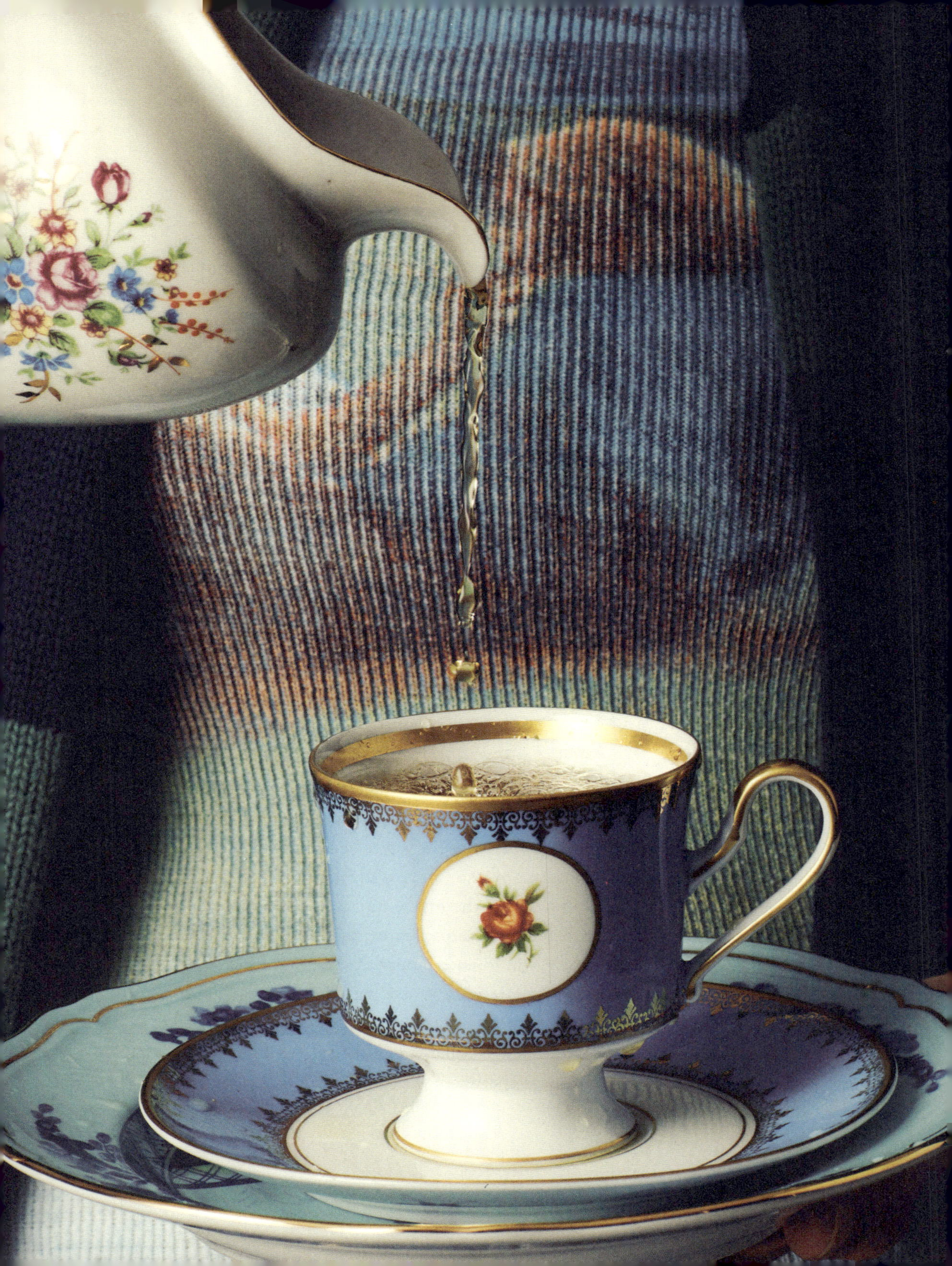

Part 1

Around the World

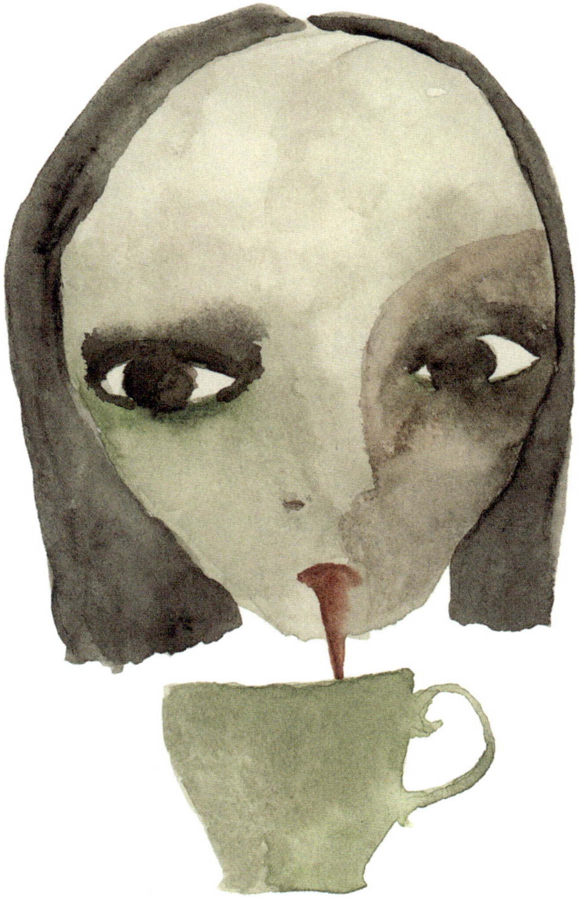

"Tea time is a talent."
— Éric Rohmer, *My Night at Maud's* (1970)

– 1 –

Tea Culture

Tea culture looks different in every corner of the world. My cultural perspective on tea is that of a New Yorker with an Eastern European lineage, a naturopathic doctor with a boutique tea company, a travel writer.

In a globalized world, drinking tea is a way to encounter cultures and a way to experience something peaceful and human as many of our ancestors did, but in a modern way. Drinking tea today can be a way to place ourselves in history, to consider what we have in common with those who came before us, and to thoughtfully place beauty at the forefront of our lives.

Tea uniquely permeates culture through films, music, and literature. Tea is a lifestyle, one which can take on many forms. For me, that lifestyle was forged through the aesthetic sensibility of New York City, summers in the country, and bike rides delivering tea for my business.

✣ ✣ ✣

To this day, one of my great unapologetic joys is drinking tea on my Brooklyn fire escape, like a twenty-one-year-old who has just arrived in New York from small-town America. Today, from my fire escape I see prayer flags blowing in the wind, I face a white brick wall, and I overlook the community garden next door. In the summer, I see ferns, the cat in my neighbor's window, and a giant hydrangea tree. A lady across the way occasionally yells obscenities out of her window. The best place to drink tea in New York City is at home. The pace of the city is a whirlwind romance, aggressive at times, magically fast. I believe that our homes in New York, small or unusual as they may be, are havens of originality, expressions of who we are at rest. It is in this setting that we can best experience the beauty of tea.

New Yorkers are from everywhere. My family is Eastern European. I was born in Kiev, Ukraine, and my parents left with me and my dad's parents in 1989, when I was nine months old, to come to New York City, where we lived until I was in third grade. Then they moved to suburban New Jersey. My grandparents stayed in Bensonhurst, Brooklyn, for the rest of their lives. Because tea culture is international, all of the people who have moved here over the years have brought their own take on it. The breadth of experience of drinking tea is widest inside of New York apartments, in people's personal collections of teaware, traditions, and comforts.

If you did not grow up drinking tea, much of what you might know about tea culture likely comes from Chinese and Japanese tea ceremonies, and for good reason. These gorgeous artistic practices are rooted in thousands of years of history and have specific rules and guidelines. Tea for Eastern Europeans embodies a different form of sophistication and ease, one that revolves around black tea, allows for mistakes in brewing, and has a looser associated methodology. Something that fascinates me is how black tea (which comes from *Camellia sinensis*, an ancient Chinese plant), has been essential enough to people and cultures throughout the world that Soviet refugees, like my family, found it important enough to bring their devices for brewing it across continents.

For me, these rituals came through my grandmother Babushka Rita and the teacups that she used. These experiences with her, both in her Brooklyn apartment and in our little bungalow in upstate New York, are my first tea memories.

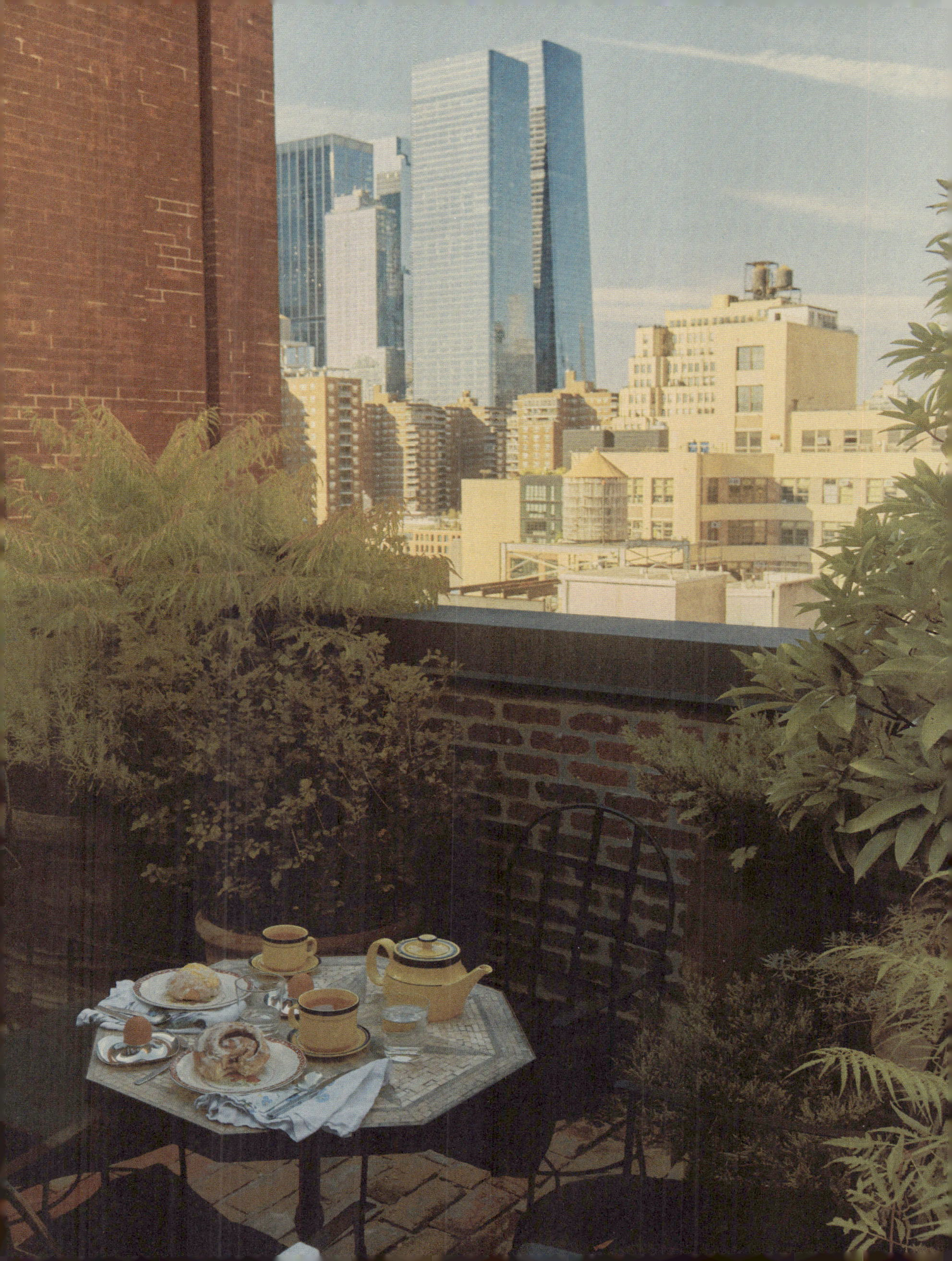

Tea with Babushka

When I was growing up, we had a bungalow in the Catskills. It was our *dacha* (summer cottage). It was a non-winterized little house with just a few rooms, a bathroom, and a netted porch. From the porch, you could see the forest on one side, woods with some houses peeking through, and our neighbor's house next door. There were four little houses on the property, including ours.

There was a little pathway in the woods where we could go on walks and pick mushrooms. My grandmother, Rita, would take a knife and a basket and we would all go looking for them. Mostly, though, my grandmother picked berries. She would cut off just the top of a gallon milk container and not leave the woods until it was full of blueberries and blackberries. Berries are something I preferred eating to picking, though there is nothing quite as satisfying as finding a giant wild blueberry bush, not yet touched, with hundreds of berries to pick clean. Because picking berries was custom for the many Eastern Europeans who spent summers in the Catskills, the trees close to roads, or near lakes, were often picked through. You really had to know where to go to find an untouched tree.

I really miss my grandmother. She was such an interesting person. She had so many stories. Most vividly, I remember her stories, told over a cup of tea. She laughed longer and louder than anyone I've ever met. It was contagious—I'm laughing as I write this—and so many things could trigger it.

Another thing about my grandmother is that she prided herself on her cooking, baking, and housekeeping skills. From sour pickles to stuffed peppers, everything was plated and served beautifully, on carefully chosen dishware, most of which she had thrifted from the flea market by her apartment in Brooklyn. She shopped at the flea market for dacha supplies for the summer: country paintings, floral dishes, sweaters, playing cards. She had a different sensibility when shopping for her Brooklyn apartment, which she filled with crystal, black and white furniture, silver clown paintings, art books, and, for her bedroom, ivory furniture, pink sheets, and thick rugs. Walls of both the apartment and the dacha were covered with art that she thrifted or that her friends made. The crystal chandelier in her Brooklyn apartment was one my dad bought for her in Prague as a gift while he was

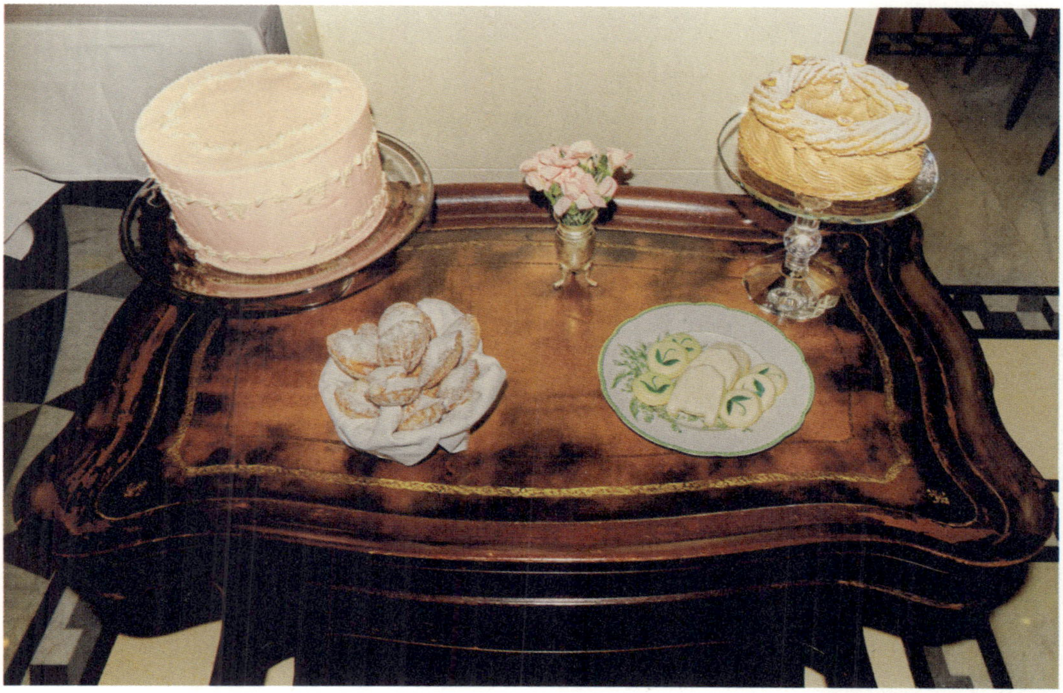

still in college. I am amazed that it made it all the way to Brooklyn during their immigration.

And of course, there was tea.

My grandmother had a primary tea set that she used in her apartment—white and pink porcelain that she brought from Kiev—and another one that lived at the dacha. She also had several tea sets that were never used but were rather part of her collection for display. She kept them in a glass case in her living room in Brooklyn. Tea was served with honey, along with snacks and desserts (see Babushka Rita's Desserts to Serve with Tea, page 133), and there was always the option to add milk or lemon to your tea, both of which were put out on the table for guests. When we stayed with her at the dacha, we drank tea three times a day: with breakfast, after lunch, and in the evening while we played cards on the porch.

Before my grandmother passed away, her apartment in Bensonhurst was my favorite place to drink tea in New York. It was a magical place to my childhood self. My parents, sister, and I would walk through the

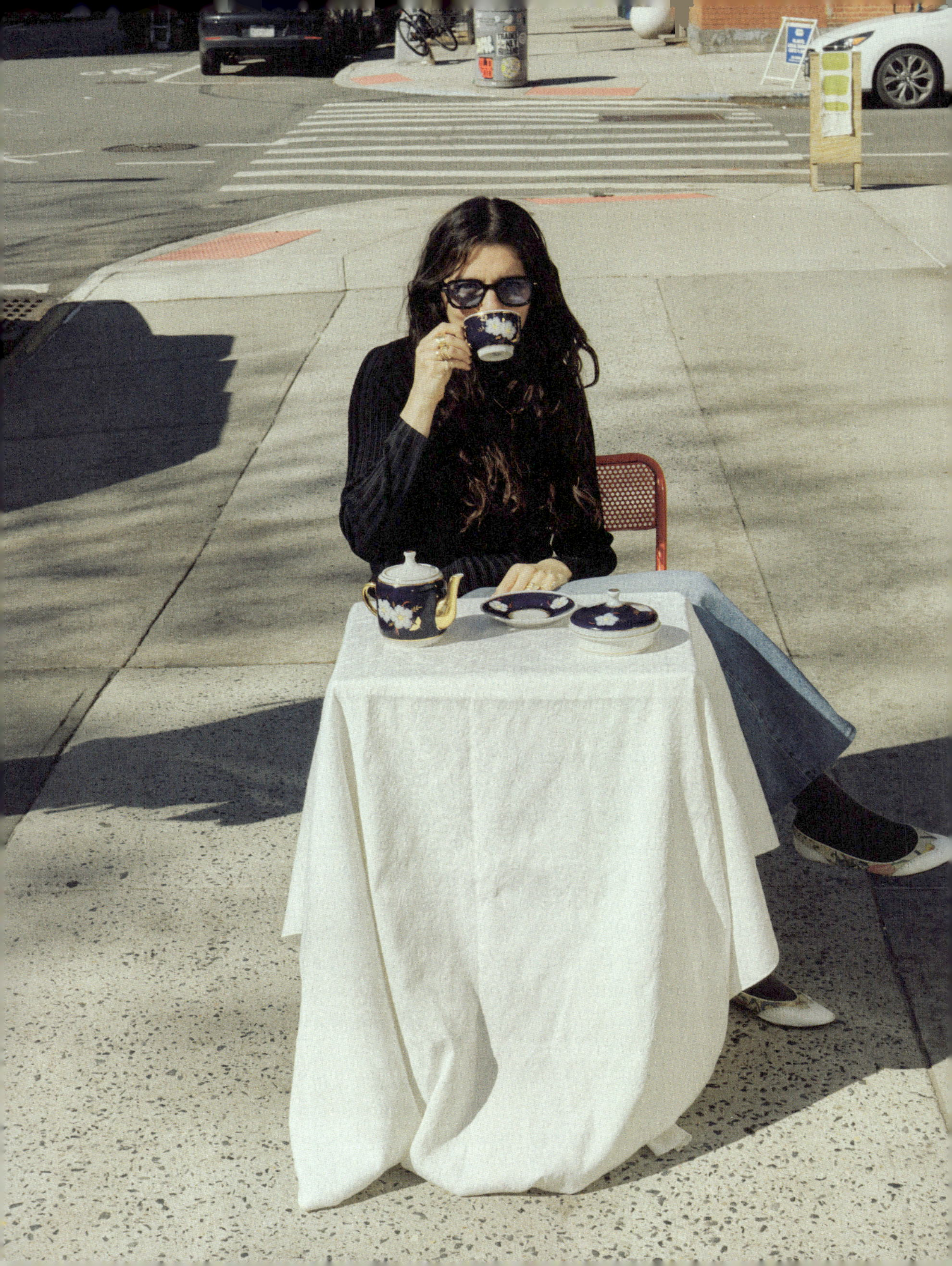

black-and-white-tiled foyer and buzz her apartment, then run in. My sister and I would head straight to her bedroom, where clothes and trinkets from the flea market were carefully laid out on her bed. Anything that we didn't choose she would pack up and send to her friends in Kiev, along with some money. Then we would all convene in the ornate living room for a spread of open-faced sandwiches, caviar, cucumbers, eggplant salad, deviled eggs, and pots of tea. If it was a special occasion, and even sometimes when it wasn't, the adults would toast with cognac. We would wait with anticipation to see which of her signature cakes would come out of the kitchen.

And so, my first experiences with tea were moments of hospitality, family, artistry, laughter, and storytelling. This was our family's tea culture and an important part of who I am.

Starting a Tea Company

When I was in high school, I no longer spent every summer upstate with my grandmother, and instead visited her in Brooklyn on weekends. Then I went to medical school, transferred to a naturopathic medical school, and eventually started a company, Masha Tea ("Masha" is the diminutive of Maria in Russian). I traveled a lot in my twenties and lived in different places, eventually moving back to Brooklyn to spend more time with my grandparents while they were still alive. While their neighborhood, Bensonhurst, remained largely unchanged, I moved to northern Brooklyn, which felt somewhat like a different world within the same borough. I started a naturopathic medical practice, where I created medicinal tea blends for my patients, and from there started packaging some of the teas and blends for my tea line.

During the Covid pandemic, in an effort to connect with people who wanted tea, I had two methods for safe tea pickups and deliveries. When customers wanted to pick up tea themselves, I would hang a basket tied with rope out of my second-floor window—like an old-world grandmother—and people would collect their tea from the basket.

I called my tea-delivery service *La Teacyclette*. I got very into cycling during the pandemic. With so few cars on the road and because many people had left the city, bike riding was actually safe. I would bike packages of matcha and other tea all over Brooklyn and Manhattan and leave them at people's doors. It was a way for me to stay healthy and create sweet relationship moments at a time when New Yorkers were perhaps most isolated from one another. Tea helped me in many ways during that particularly stressful time. Drinking tea calmed me down, but also getting tea to other New Yorkers, through these bike deliveries and also by selling tea at the farmers markets every weekend, enabled me to be a part of the community and connected me with people seeking similar rituals.

The Aesthetics of Tea

Tea is multisensorial: the smell of tea leaves, color in a cup, and the sound of water pouring create a visceral experience, which is why tea is strongly tied to memory. Artists highlight this—in paintings, film, and literature—often adding tea scenes to create intimacy or to give a sense of what the character has been up to before the current scene.

Start looking for tea scenes while watching movies and you will see them, discreetly, everywhere. A maid pouring tea in the foreground while two of the main characters are having a conversation, lovers meeting for a tryst, a teapot and cups in the background. Read classic literature—Russian, English, and Japanese—and you will find characters congregating over tea. Because drinking tea is lovely and cinematic, it is inherently part of a life well lived, just like a well-lit room to read in, a perfectly fitting dress, or a waterfall. That is the aesthetic aspect of tea.

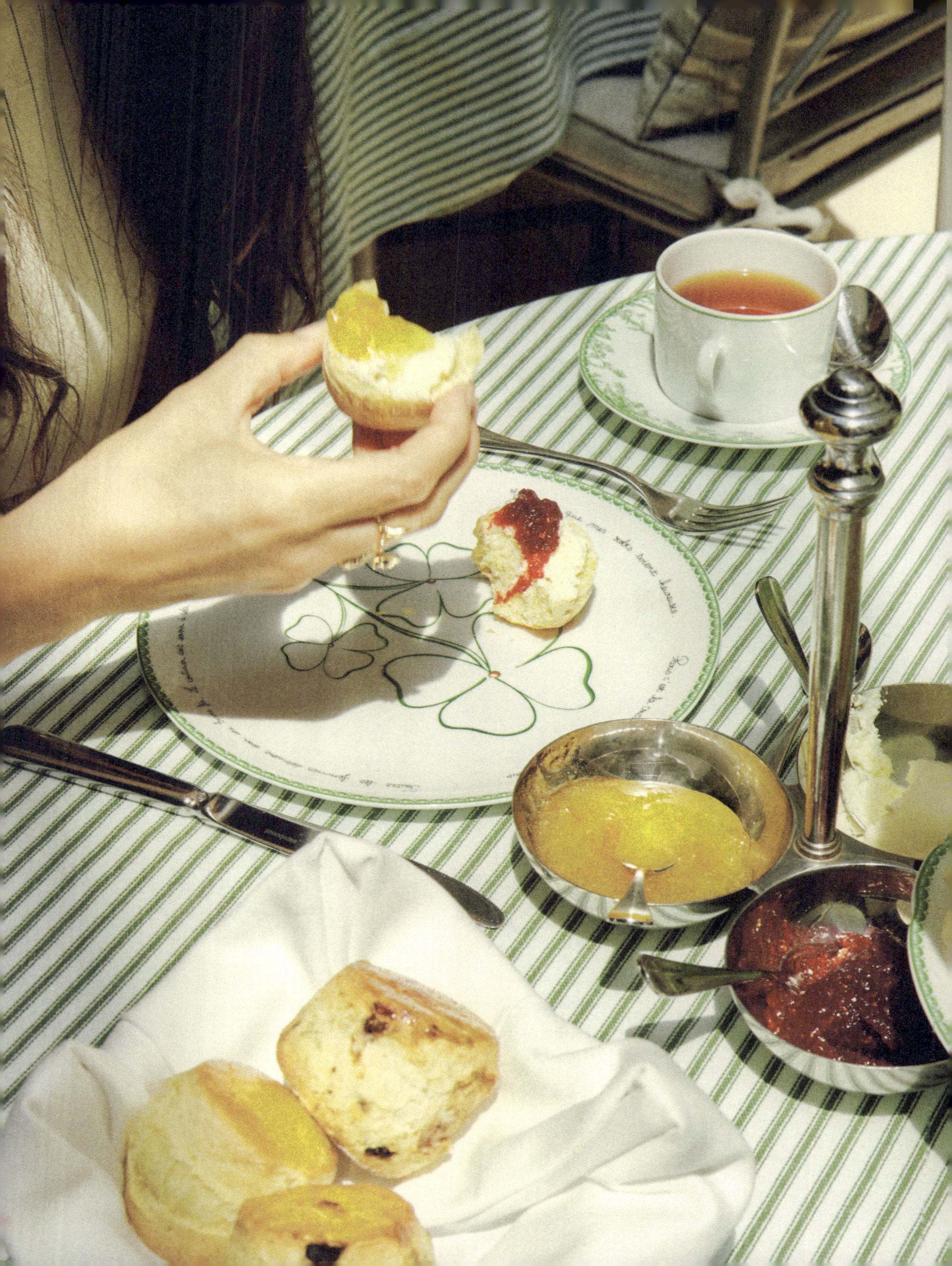

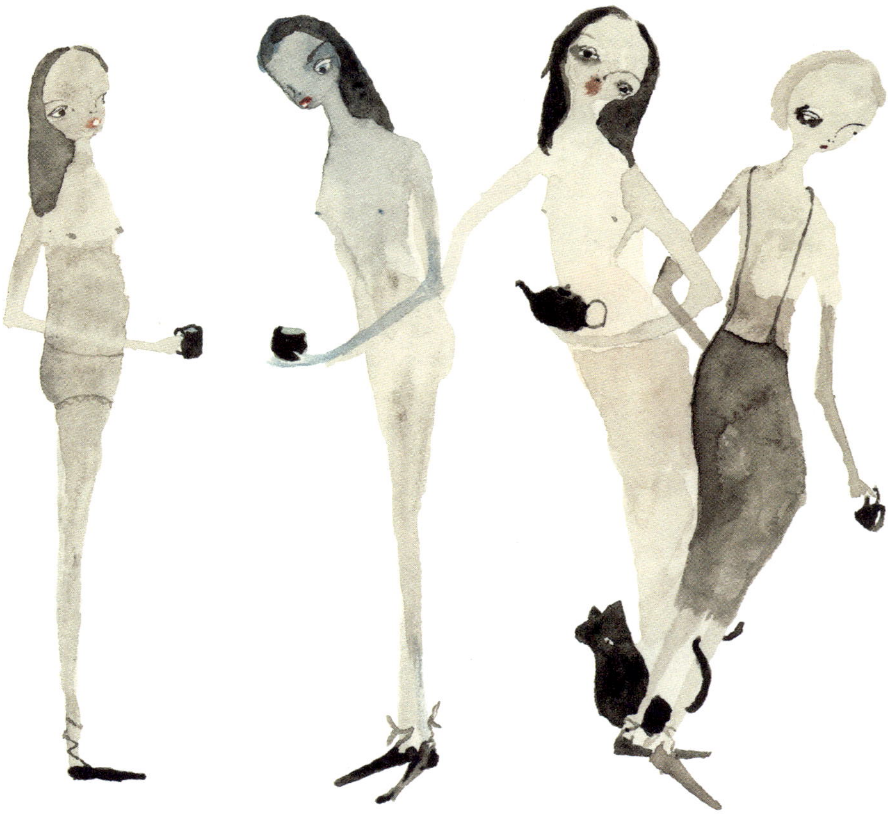

"The effect of tea is cooling and as a beverage it is most suitable. It is especially fitting for persons of self-restraint and inner worth."
—Lu Yu, *The Classic of Tea* (780 AD)

– 2 –

Tea on Planet Earth: Stories and Myths

When it comes to events that took place thousands of years ago, history blurs into myth. Even as cycles repeat, it is easy to feel removed from history, bored by the details. But there are through lines—experiences so innately human that we've done them seemingly forever as a species. Drinking tea is such an experience. Besides evidence of humans boiling tea in water three hundred thousand years ago, during the Paleolithic Period, tea has been a part of modern history for over three thousand years. Imagine having tea and a conversation with a friend or coworker, commenting that the tea is too hot and still needs a moment to cool. This type of observational small talk has persisted across languages, centuries, and geographical borders.

Tea has been transported on camels, horses, ships, and airplanes. Tea has been a tool for negotiation and used as an instigator for conflict, a plant indigenous to China and India that is now practically ubiquitous in kitchens the world over. The stories and myths in the coming pages specifically refer to *Camellia sinensis,* the tea plant from which green, black, white, oolong, and pu'erh teas are all made. Though later in this book I refer to various herbs as tea, this chapter on tea history and legends refers specifically to *Camellia sinensis.* The Latin *Camellia sinensis* comes from *Camellia,* an allusion to Georg Joseph Kamel, a priest and botanist, and *sinensis,* meaning "from China."

Caravan Tea:
Tea Culture in Eastern Europe

As someone who came from Eastern Europe, I will start this tea history there. I was born in Kiev, now Ukraine, at the time a part of the Soviet Union, and my grandparents and parents left with me when I was nine months old. The path out of the Soviet Union for Jewish refugees at the time was to formally state that you were leaving for Israel, but ultimately decide where you wanted to land once in Europe. My family was always set on New York City. When my dad spoke of Ukraine and Russia, he would sometimes explain to me that this region of the world was a point of tension, never at peace because it's a confluence of the East and West.

The tea trade and paths taken to transport tea tell a version of the globalization story—tea was one of the original incentives for—and objects of—trade in a globalizing world. Kyakhta in Russia and Canton in China were the two cities most central to global trade before the Chinese Opium Wars in the mid-1800s. Tea carried to Kyakhta from Kalgan, China, by camels or oxen carts through the desert was called "caravan tea." In contrast, tea shipped from Canton, China, to London and then distributed around Europe (some of which went to Russia as well) was called "Canton tea."

Caravan tea was considered higher quality than Canton: the long overseas voyage diminished the tea quality, whereas the desert climate on the caravan tea route was said to enhance the flavor of the tea. Chinyun Lee writes in, "From Kiachta to Vladivostok: Russian Merchants and the Tea Trade": During the winter, 50,000 camels carried caravan tea from Kalgan, outside the Great Wall, to Kiachta. From there, it was transported by [sleigh] to fairs throughout Siberia.

Russian tea was usually enjoyed black, with black bread and occasionally with vodka, so the taste of the tea was paramount. In Britain, where tea was always served with milk, the strength of the tea mattered more than the taste. Later in Russia, when cheaper teas were imported from colonial India, they were harvested to be strong rather than refined.

Sergei Iul'evich Witte became the Imperial Russian minister of finance in 1882, at which time construction of the Trans-Siberian Railroad began and eventually rerouted sea transport from Shanghai to Vladivostok. (Tea was sent to Vladivostok, the easternmost origin of the Trans-Siberian Railroad, and could be transported to Moscow from there.) In a memorandum to Tsar Alexander III, Witte listed the economic benefits of the railroad project, including "assisting China in her rivalry with England in the tea market, and gain[ing] Chinese support for Russia with regard to England." The railroads would expedite the tea deliveries when compared to the glamorous yet arduous use of camels. Russian demand for Chinese tea continued to grow. Eventually, Russia also began using cheaper import routes over the seas. From the late 1800s until World War I, Russia and England competed for the finite supply of Chinese tea. During World War I, the Russian government bought enormous quantities of tea for the army. The peak came in 1915, when over seventy thousand tons of tea were ordered.

Russian imports of Chinese tea ultimately ended with the Bolshevik Revolution of 1917, when the government ended diplomatic relations with China.

The Soviet government decided to invest in its own tea cultivation in Georgia, promoting the Soviet principle of self-sufficiency. Ultimately, the region never grew enough tea to eliminate the need for foreign imports (the tea plant requires at least five years of cultivation to reach a commercial level of production).

The sourcing of tea changed again in the 1950s, when China entered the Communist bloc and a trade agreement formed between India and the Soviet Union, leading the latter to begin importing large quantities of both Indian and Chinese tea.

By the 1980s, when my parents were in their twenties, the more affordable, and more accessible, tea in Soviet stores was probably the Indian variety. They coveted Sri Lankan tea as well.

As a Soviet-immigrant family, when I was growing up we mostly drank Indian black tea. When I went to college and visited the Russian stores in Bensonhurst and Brighton Beach, where my grandparents and aunt and uncle lived, and even the Russian stores in New Jersey near my parents' house, I loved buying a loose tea called Czar Nicholai II: Russian Caravan. It must have been that Chinese style of tea.

Tea Culture in China

The story goes that the legendary Chinese emperor Shen Nung stopped to rest under a tree. According to custom, he boiled water before drinking it. Suddenly, a leaf from a nearby tea tree fell and floated down into his cup. Intrigued, he watched the water change color and upon drinking it, felt a profound sense of calm. This moment, about three thousand years ago, would change the course of China's history, and eventually, world history.

Along with discovering tea, Shen Nung pioneered the system of traditional Chinese medicine through his studies of the medicinal properties of hundreds of plants and his creation of the system of acupuncture. Because of Shen Nung, the use of tea as a form of medicine began; this tradition would continue for centuries to come.

Another tea origin story also takes place in China, but it features an Indian prince, the Buddhist monk Bodhidharma. Bodhidharma arrived in China around 470 AD to reintroduce Buddhism to the country. The legend goes that he vowed to spend nine years in meditation without sleeping and the tea plant itself sprung from his tired eyelids. By drinking tea, he was able to continue his meditation and stay awake, completing his vow.

Wild tea plants in China grew quite tall and farmers simply cut them down to access the leaves. However, they realized there was a danger of overharvesting. And so, in the fourth century, farmers began cultivating tea plants rather than simply sourcing them wild from forests. Tea plants love well-drained soil, so from the beginning, tea has mostly been planted on hillsides.

Originally, people in China prepared tea by boiling the leaves with rice, ginger, salt, citrus peels, milk, spices, and onions. Tea-growing and tea-processing styles and customs became increasingly refined until great tea was meant to be enjoyed on its own. People opened teahouses and began to write about tea. Lu Yu wrote *Ch'a Ching* (*The Classic of Tea*) in 780 AD, a three-volume, ten-chapter book on everything one needs to know about the tea cultivation and tea drinking of the time.

China's neighbors began to covet tea, and it was traded for horses (through what was known as the Tea and Horse Caravan Road). Later, tea consumption spread to Korea and Japan through Buddhism.

Tea Culture in Japan

"Teaism is a cult founded on the adoration of the beautiful among the sordid facts of everyday existence."
—Kakuzō Okakura, *The Book of Tea* (1906)

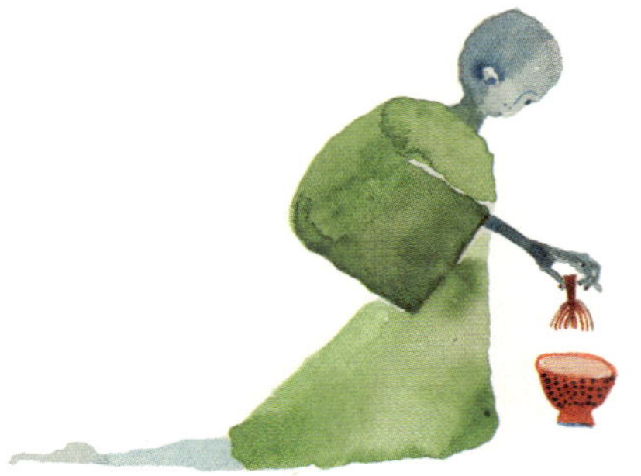

In the twelfth century, after studying Zen Buddhism in China, Japanese monks returned to their home country with tea seeds. After hundreds of years, Zen Buddhist principles such as simplicity (*kanso*), naturalness (*shizen*), and tranquility (*seijaku*) became essential elements in Japanese tea culture. The Japanese tea ceremony, called *Chanoyu* in Japan, is a structured ritual with a specific set of tools and rules for host and guest alike. The ceremony, first started by tea master Sen no Rikyū in the sixteenth century, contains elements of drama, flowers, paintings, conversation, and beauty. Because of the strong Zen Buddhist roots, pillars of Zen translated to the tearoom.

The descriptions used for Japanese tearooms (*sukiyas*) are described as ideographs—words that represent abstract ideas, leaving them open to interpretation (*liberty*, *democracy*, and *justice* are ideographs in English). In the Japanese written language, ideographs, or *kanji*, similar to Chinese *hanzi*, are the characters that represent concepts rather than sounds. So, with the example of *sukiya*, the tearoom first meant "abode of fancy," though it could also signify "abode of vacancy" or "abode of the unsymmetrical."

The Japanese teahouse is itself intentionally structured: a room fitting no more than five people, a front room for washing and arranging tea utensils, a garden path, and a waiting room for guests.

As tea became more prevalent in Japan, the culture and ceremony became traditionalized but continued to evolve. In a similar spirit to bringing in tea through Chinese Buddhism, scholars believe that the Japanese may have integrated aesthetic elements of the Catholic Mass, which European priests brought to Japan in the sixteenth century, to the tea ceremony. The cup being lifted high and wiped clean with a cloth, for example, is seen in both the Catholic Mass and the Japanese tea ceremony. With tea, Japan took a Chinese plant and, in all ways, created one of the world's strongest and most iconic tea cultures.

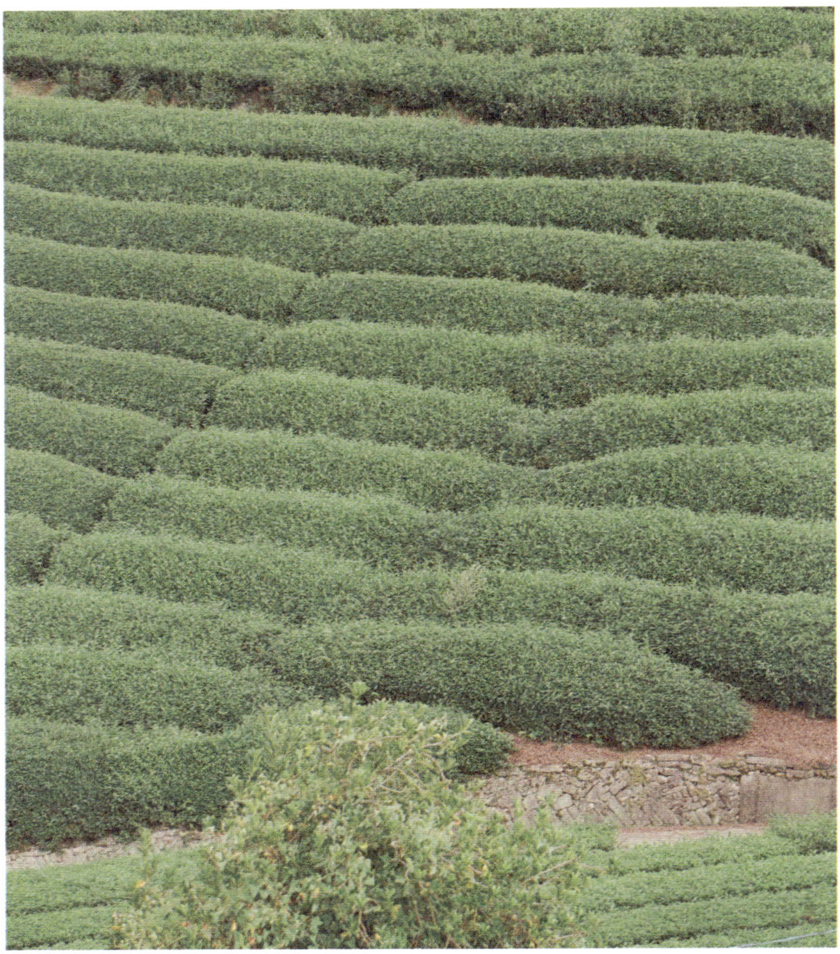

Tea Culture in India

"Come oh come ye tea-thirsty restless ones—the kettle boils, bubbles and sings, musically."
—Rabindranath Tagore

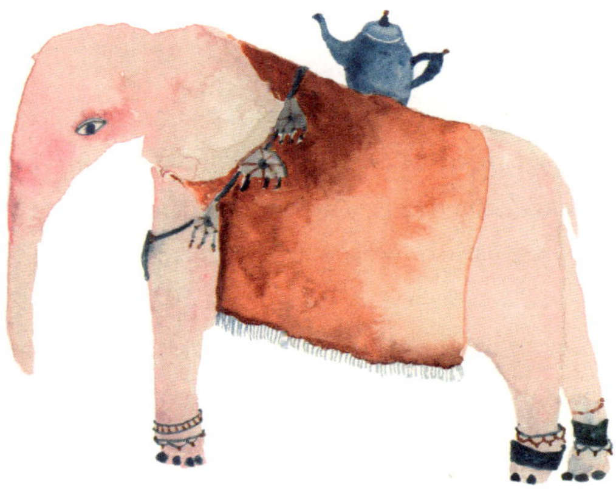

You can't dive into the world of tea without considering the history of colonialism, and that is especially true when examining how British demand for tea impacted colonial India. In the late 1600s, King Charles II married Portuguese princess and avowed tea lover Catherine of Braganza, popularizing the drink in England. The British East India Company gained a monopoly on trade in China and India at that time, leading England to make fortunes trading tea and eventually integrating it into British culture across class.

Modern tea culture in India began during the colonial period. British demand for tea exceeded the capacity of China's production capabilities. Due to China's monopoly, cost was quite high. The British eventually stole tea plants and tea-growing techniques from China in what became known as "the Great Tea Heist," which involved sending a Scottish botanist named Robert Fortune in disguise to China. By successfully stealing both tea seeds and the knowledge of how to cultivate them, Fortune (aptly named) profoundly, though maliciously, impacted the course of tea history by recognizing a healthy tea-growing environment in India.

Camellia sinensis var. assamica, the strain of tea growing wild in the Assam region of North India, was also identified and found to be quite similar to Chinese tea. Local people drank tea in this region for centuries, but it was this commercial demand that led to the formation of large-scale tea farming. Tea farms and gardens, of both Chinese native *Camellia sinensis var. sinensis* and Indian native *Camellia sinensis var. assamica,* were cultivated over huge stretches of India, first in northern India in Darjeeling and Assam, but later in southern states as well.

While *Camellia sinensis var. assamica* was not cultivated or consumed on a mass scale prior to colonization, herbal teas were cultivated in Ayurvedic gardens and consumed throughout India for millennia.

Today, India is most known for its black teas (though green, oolong, and white teas are now produced in the country). Though originally tea was considered a symbol of imperialism, thus unattractive to Indian people, in the early twentieth century there was such an abundance of tea in India that producers began marketing tea domestically, first to the upper classes. There was a long-standing history of drinking spices in milk in India, from thousands of years of Ayurvedic tradition. By the 1930s, Indian people across classes were drinking domestically grown tea. Rather than steeping it in water, black tea was boiled in milk and water with spices like ginger, cardamom, black pepper, and clove to make the now-classic Indian beverage, chai, which translates simply to tea.

Tea cultivation continued in post-colonial India and tea sales, both domestically and abroad, continue to be a major source of revenue for the country. India and China are the world's two largest tea-producing countries today. There are countless recipes for chai across India, with spices varying depending on which part of the country you are in and even within households. While Indian chai can refer most simply to tea with milk and sugar, masala chai always includes spices. Another version, Irani chai, involves simmering the milk slowly and at length, separately from the black tea and sugar, then combining what is a resulting condensed-milk-like preparation, with or without spices, to the tea just before serving. What was once a symbol of colonialism became something quintessentially Indian.

Tea Culture in North America

In the late 1700s, for the first time, an American trade ship, the *Empress of China,* sailed from New York to Canton, China, with hundreds of barrels of *Panax quinquefolius,* colloquially known as American ginseng, a plant indigenous to the Appalachian Mountains. There was high demand for it in China for its use in Traditional Chinese Medicine as an alternative to Asian ginseng. In turn, China traded a plant that was indigenous there: tea. This journey marked the beginning of America's entry into tea trade, which was once monopolized by Britain's East India Company. Of the trip, Philip Freneau, "poet of the American Revolution," wrote:

> She now her eager course explores,
> And soon shall meet Chinesian shores,
> From thence their fragrant TEAS to bring
> Without the leave of Britain's king;
> And PORCELAIN WARE, enchased in gold,
> The product of that finer mould.

So began a trading partnership that was enriching for the several Americans who were favored by Houqua, a Chinese millionaire and one of the richest men in the world at the time. The multimillion-dollar tea trade helped mint some of America's first millionaires by creating a demand for fast ships that could sail back and forth from China.

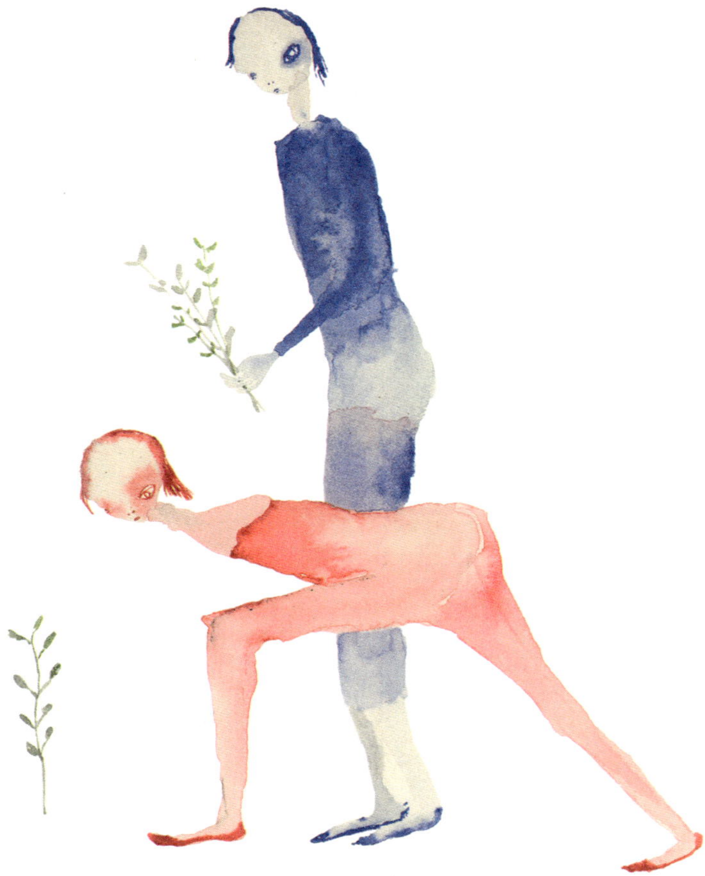

"Birds, beasts, and men all exist between heaven and earth and rely upon food and drink to sustain life. How mysterious is the reality of drinking. One quenches thirst by drinking water, one dispels anxiety by drinking wine, and to banish sleep and raise alertness, one must drink tea."
—Lu Yu, *The Classic of Tea* (780 AD)

– 3 –

Tea and Herb Farms

Something that many a tea lover will tell you is that the enjoyment of a cup of tea depends greatly on the context in which you are drinking it: the teaware used, music playing, clothing worn, and scents around you all impact the experience. These aesthetic details, along with sustainability and equity considerations, such as sourcing teas that ensure fair wages for local farm workers, and sourcing herbs locally, when possible, versus from abroad, inform the storytelling and world of Masha Tea. With tea, elements of artistry exist in both growing tea and drinking it. Tea is not inanimate, but rather a result of thoughtful human decisions—from design to agriculture.

It is possible to create a tea-like beverage using local plants anywhere in the world. In New York City, farmers markets sell herbs grown in our region, and many of us grow herbs on balconies, rooftops, or community gardens. Opt for local when possible, from a supplier that you trust. When that's not possible, look for organic and fair-trade teas. If traveling to a region of the world where tea grows, there is nothing as memorable as sitting on a mountainside overlooking a tea plantation.

Globally, pesticide use in farming began with industrialization. Before pesticides, all farms were organic. Organic farming today refers to a natural style of agriculture that favors crop rotation, beneficial insects, and biodiversity. At a time when pesticides are being linked to cancer, immunotoxicity, and reproductive issues, and soil health is being depleted from monocropping, organic farming practices are widely considered healthier. Because industrial farming has globalized over the past century, returning to natural ways of growing food—and in this case tea—is often more expensive and smaller scale. Some farms grow organic but cannot afford certification and forgo it. I only source teas that are grown organically.

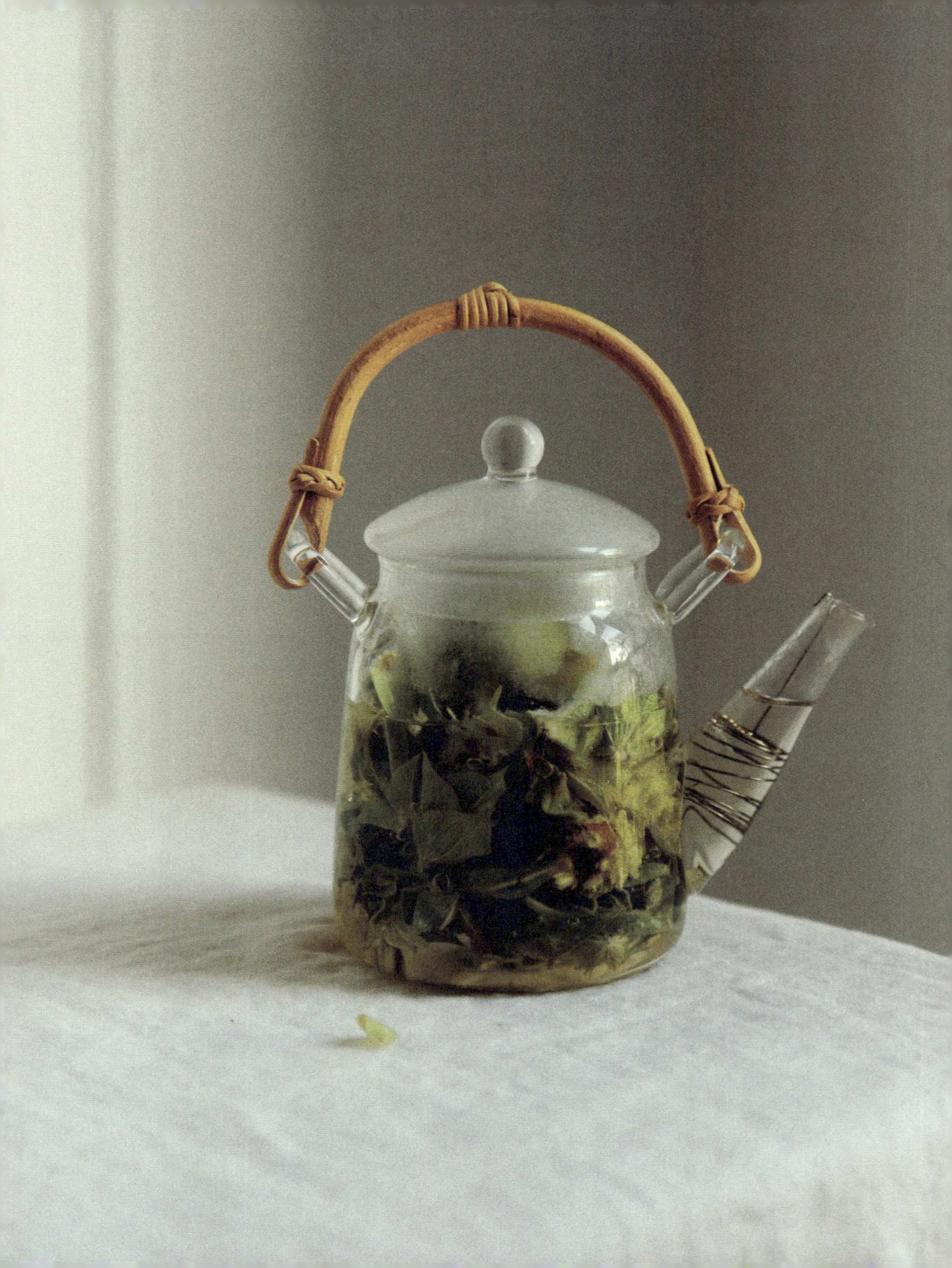

What Tea Is and Where It Grows

Tea is a drink made from steeping herbs in water. Black, green, white, oolong, and pu'erh all come from the tea plant, *Camellia sinensis*, but there are a range of plants that can be used to make teas. Herbal teas, or tisanes, can be made from the leaves, stems, roots, and flowers of a plant. Grains such as barley, rice, and buckwheat also make delicious teas, as do mushrooms.

When it comes to medicinal plants, the herbs in question are sometimes considered weeds. I think it's important to reframe the idea of a weed. A plant so resilient that it can grow in cracks in sidewalks or overgrow gardens shows strength and power that can often be harnessed medicinally, as tea or otherwise.

High-quality tea, no matter the type, is something growing, alive, and vibrant that was produced by the artisanal care of the people who farm, process, and package it into what you have at home. Because there are so many steps between growth and tea leaves (or bags), people don't often make the connection of what tea truly is and where it comes from: soil, water, sun, human hands. Seasonality, which we normally attribute to vegetables and fruits, is something that is applicable in the world of tea as well. Seasonality in tea applies to ideal harvesttime. Some plants have a short window—cherry blossoms bloom for just a few weeks in spring, wild rose buds bloom in early summer, spruce tips in spring, and wild chamomile in mid-summer. The tea plant, too, is tied to seasonality, as it's harvested from spring into fall.

Tea is grown the world over: yerba maté in South America, specifically Argentina, Brazil, Paraguay, and Uruguay; Greek mountain tea in Greece; rooibos in South Africa. There is hibiscus tea from Mexico, mint tea from Turkey, and white tea from Indonesia. This book focuses on the places that have been pertinent to my humble, personal experience: the countries where I have sourced tea for my company and have visited in my travels.

Tea in Japan

"Meanwhile, let us have a sip of tea. The afternoon glow is brightening the bamboos, the fountains are bubbling with delight, the soughing of the pines is heard in our kettle. Let us dream of evanescence and linger in the beautiful foolishness of things."
—Kakuzō Okakura, *The Book of Tea* (1906)

✧ ✧ ✧

Tea farming and tea culture began in Japan because of Buddhism. Zen Buddhism originated in India, spread to China, and eventually took root in eighth-century Japan. At that time, both Chinese and Japanese cultures drank brick tea, a style wherein the tea is hard pressed together into a "brick" and then a small amount is scraped off and brewed with boiled water. Around the twelfth century, powdered green tea, now known as matcha, was introduced to Japan from China. Though matcha was originally cultivated in China, it lost popularity there in part due the fourteenth-century Hongwu Emperor's ban on compressed tea; he sought to simplify labor related to tea production and shifted the country toward loose tea. Matcha became refined in Japan and is now considered a defining symbol of Japanese tea culture and ceremony. I have visited tea farms to source tea in Uji and in Shizuoka, one of Japan's oldest and largest green tea–growing regions, on the south side of Mount Fuji. Along with Shizuoka and Uji, an important center of both green and matcha tea culture in Japan is in the seaside former capital, Kamakura.

While tea was first brought to Japan in the eighth century, it flourished in twelfth-century Japan, during the Kamakura period, when Eisie, a Japanese Buddhist priest responsible for spreading Zen to his home country, brought tea seeds to Kamakura from China. I stayed at a modern *ryokan* (inn) in Kamakura, Kishi-ke, with a strong focus on tea ceremony influenced by the Zen history of the region. The proprietor created the space based around the Zen principle of *chisoku*, which loosely translates to "being satisfied with what you already have." And it does appear easy to be satisfied

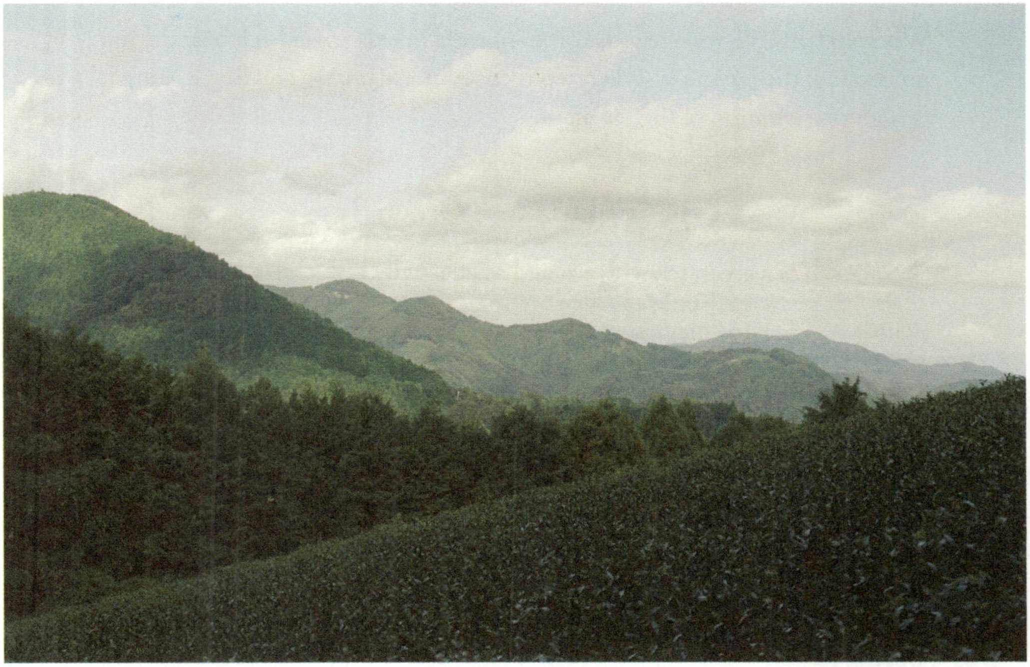

with what you have there: Through the front window lies a straight-on view of surfers in the ocean, fashionable cars rolling along the coastal road, and sailboats in the far distance. In the backyard is a private Zen garden, and, on the inside, meticulous interiors featuring a generously sized traditional Hinoki bath—a wooden tub made of Hinoki cypress wood—and a vast ceramics collection.

I must have used dozens of different cups over the course of my long-weekend stay, ranging from pieces repaired using *kintsugi*—a way of fixing broken pottery using gold dust (see page 72)—to matcha bowls made from volcanic rock from Mount Fuji and dainty, translucent white cups. Along with classic Japanese teas like matcha and hōjicha, I had teas that I'd never tried before like blueberry leaf and *goishicha*, which translates to "square stone tea," a rare lacto-fermented tea grown only in Ôtoyo in Kôchi Prefecture. The flavor is slightly sour and mushroomy at the same time.

While cultivation of tea in Japan at the onset mimicked that of Chinese growing practices, Japanese tea farming transformed into its own tradition.

Whereas Chinese-style teas are often roasted in woks over high heat during processing, the Japanese style often focuses on steaming, creating a gentler, fresher presentation of the tea plant.

Types of Japanese Green Teas

GENMAICHA: a green tea with toasted rice; usually kukicha is used.

HŌJICHA: a roasted green tea; tastes toasty, usually kukicha is used.

KUKICHA: also called "twig tea," this cutting of the tea includes the stems.

MATCHA: shade-grown green tea milled into a fine powder.

SENCHA: a classic of green tea leaves.

TENCHA: shade-grown green tea used for making matcha.

In Japan, most tea farms are conventional, versus organic, so it took some digging to find the small farms that I now work with to source our organic teas and matcha. For something as healthy, simple, and pure as tea, I find it important to use the most naturally grown versions of the plant.

Tea in India

I visited India for the first time when I was twenty years old. I was there for a spring semester studying abroad at a tiny secular ashram called Fireflies on the outskirts of Bangalore in South India.

Bangalore is an enormous city. There's an industrial center, but the outskirts are quite rural and there are tiny villages that are part of Bangalore proper. Fireflies was in one of these villages, Dinnepalya. I was there with nine other students from my small public liberal arts college in New Jersey and our program focused on sustainability and ecology. We took breaks for tea and cookies twice a day, in addition to having tea with every meal. My first visit to a tea farm was on that trip. We would take trips as a group around Karnataka (the state where Bangalore is located), but also to neighboring Kerala and Tamil Nadu.

It was on one such trip, through the mountains, where there were green rolling hills with tea growing on them as far as the eye could see. I remember riding on the trains in India and every hour or so, a vendor would come down the aisle shouting COFFEE, CHAI, COFFEE, CHAI, COFFEE, CHAI. On long drives, I remember the roadside tea stands serving that classic sweet, milky chai in metal cups. The chai in South India wasn't as spicy as in North India—just milk, sugar, and black tea. In North India, the chai blends include herbs like ginger, cardamom, clove, black pepper, and, of course, milk and sugar.

Types of Indian Tea

CHAI: Indian-style chai is thick with milk and sugar. It's often as much spice as it is tea. Cardamom, ginger, black pepper, cinnamon, clove, star anise, and fennel are all ground to a powder and cooked with milk, sugar, and black tea.

CTC: "Crush, Tear, and Curl" machines cut up tea leaves and make them cheaper, stronger, and easier to put in tea bags. The size and quick brewing time of these tea leaves also makes them ideal for making chai, as it's still possible to taste the black tea despite the heaviness of the milk and sugar.

FAIR TRADE: When choosing teas from India, look for fair-trade certification, which ensures that the people behind the product are being paid and treated fairly, with decent working conditions.

NORTH INDIA: Darjeeling is considered the highest quality and makes a lovely amber tea. Assam can come from both indigenous varieties, *Camellia sinensis var. assamica*, and the cultivated *Camellia sinensis var. sinsensis.*

SOUTH INDIA: Tamil Nadu, Kerala, and Karnataka are the three states where most black tea farms are found.

Tea in Italy

I took my first steps on a sandy beach in coastal Italy. There's a photo of it, with my grandmother running out of the frame in her bathing suit. Since then, I've returned to Italy many times. I love Italy. It's hot and colorful, and the people are so gracious and funny.

I have friend who converted his family home in Tuscany into a retreat center and a working organic olive oil farm. I went there for the first time on a retreat as the on-site naturopathic doctor. I would have a session with each guest in exchange for my stay. Years later, I started hosting my own tea and writing retreats there. I still host these some summers—completely unstructured, they're just a place to not have to do anything aside from coming together for meals. I bring Masha Tea, notebooks, and pens for the guests.

I remembered the abundant wildflowers from my first time on the farm. The poppies and fields of chamomile flowers. I now source chamomile every year from my friend's farm. The herbs that grow wild in Italy—lavender, mint, licorice, chamomile—are so aromatic and gentle for tea. Many of these plants grow throughout Europe and are part of the Western herbalist tradition, and they also grow well in our climate.

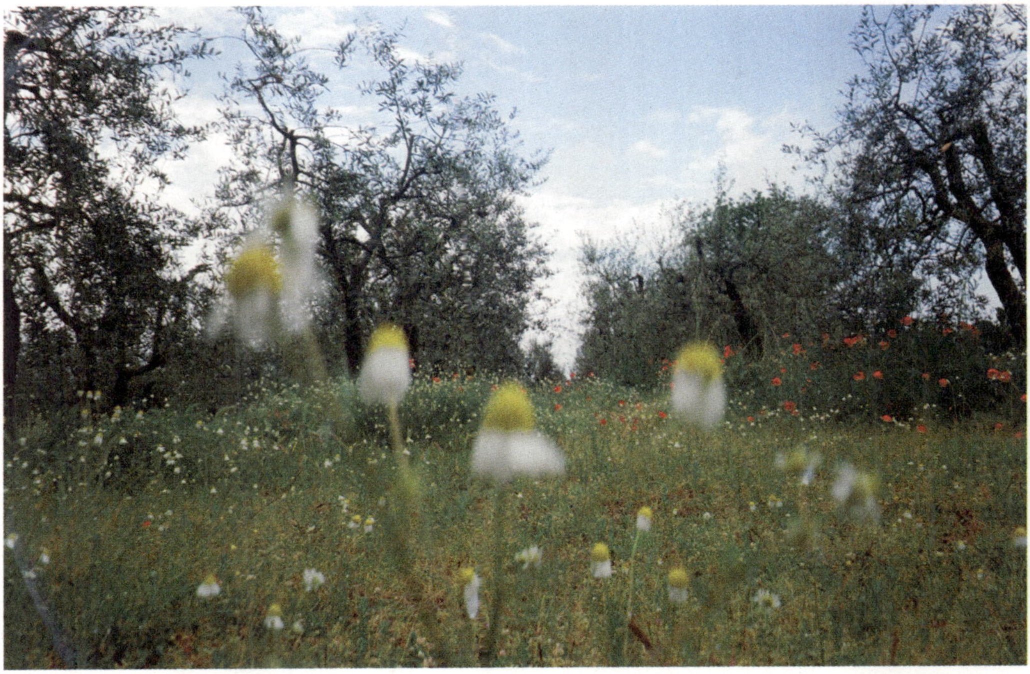

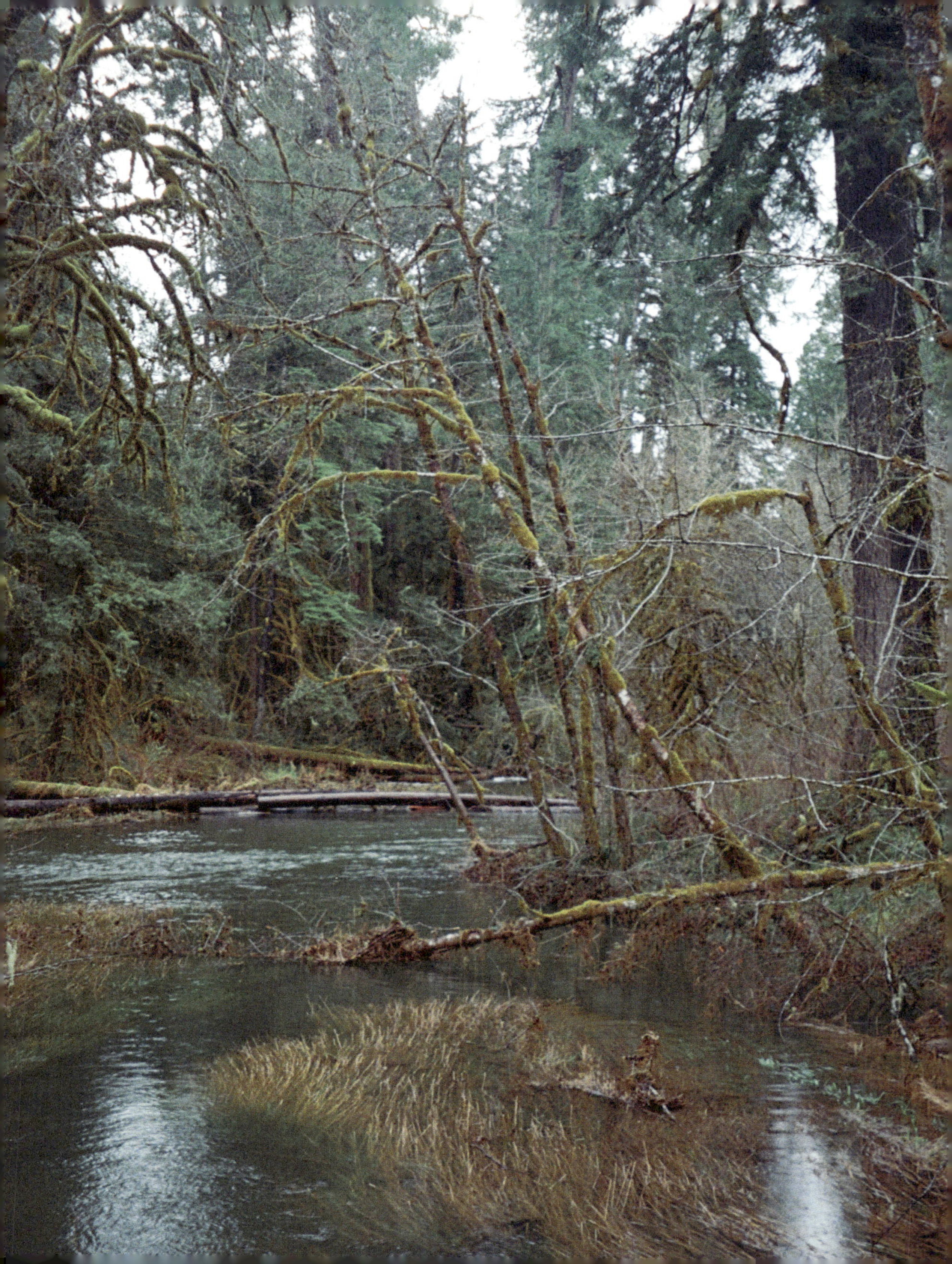

Tea in the U.S.

One of the distinguishing characteristics of Masha Tea, as compared to other tea purveyors, is the focus on sourcing herbs grown in the United States. I have visited Long Island, Vermont, and Oregon farms, and I have sourced wild-harvested herbs from trips to Wyoming, Washington State, and the Catskills. Many of these herbs and plants have been used medicinally by Native Americans and exist only in this landscape. Others grow both in the U.S. and in Europe due to their similar climates, and still others were brought in from other parts of the world over time. Herbs grow everywhere, and many of them are quite resilient and can grow under unfavorable conditions, so whether you live in the desert of New Mexico or the mountains in Alaska, it is possible to make tea from local herbs. The focus for me and my tea company has been mostly herbs grown in the Northeast and Pacific Northwest, though there are dozens of desert herbs that grow in the Southwest, and flowers and citrus from California or Florida that could apply here as well.

Pacific Northwest

Much of the bioregion in the Pacific Northwest, namely Oregon and Washington, is temperate rainforest, with gushing waterfalls, lush greenery from the long rainy season, and volcanic soil. The progressive spirit of the region makes it a hub of alternative and complementary medicine and some of the first and largest herb farms in the country. In addition to growing local herbs, Portland, where I lived for years during graduate school, is a great tea city, home to several successful tea companies and several tea gardens.

Northeast

On the East Coast, I've sourced herbs like nettle from tiny farms on the North Fork of Long Island, mint from the Catskills, chamomile from slightly larger farms in Appalachia, and tulsi from Vermont.

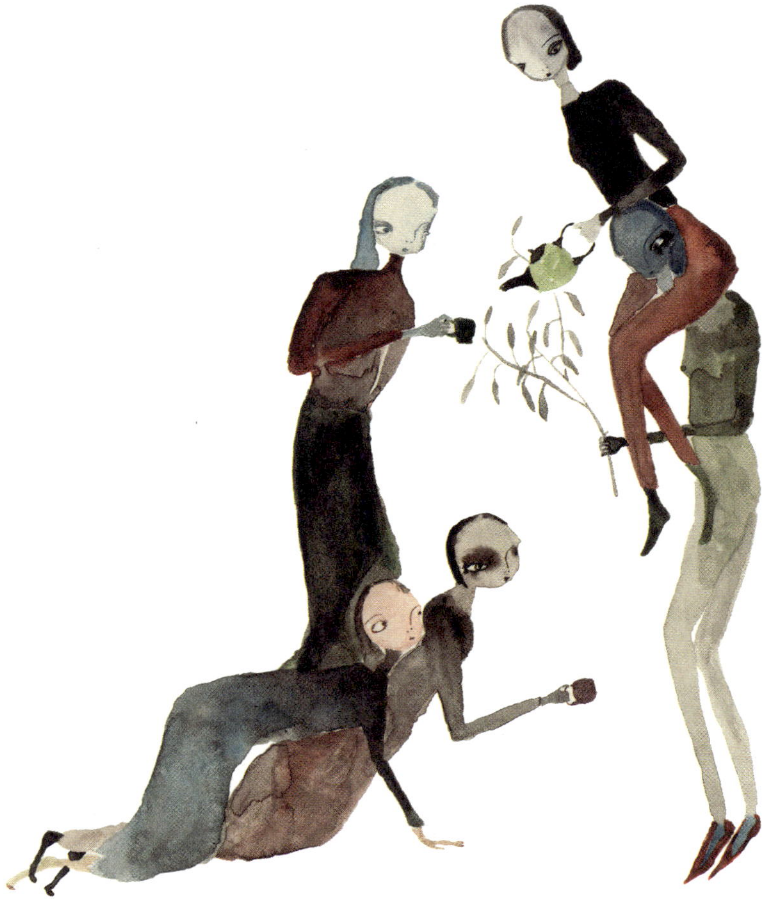

"Japhy got out the tea, Chinese tea, and sprinkled some in a tin pot, and had the fire going meanwhile, a small one to begin with, the sun was still on us, and stuck a long stick tight down under a few big rocks and made himself something to hang the teapot on and pretty soon the water was boiling and he poured it out steaming into the tin pot and we had cups of tea with our tin cups."

—Jack Kerouac, *The Dharma Bums* (1958)

– 4 –

Tea and Travel

Traveling with tea as a focus involves a particular sensibility. While somebody who loves fashion may always look to the streets to see what people are wearing, for interesting color combinations and beloved silhouettes, a tea lover looks for a teapot styled in a window, for the cake shop that carries delicious tea pairings, or the antique store with lovely vintage tea accoutrements like linens and spoons. A tea lover learns about the tea culture of a region to understand which teas and herbs grow locally, how local people take their tea—spiced or with milk for example—and the history of tea that influenced contemporary tea culture. Choosing a book for your trip that takes place in the setting where you're going, and watching movies that take place there, are other opportunities to deepen your understanding of tea's importance to a travel destination.

I always bring tea with me when I travel, but where I'm going determines how much. If I'm going somewhere luxurious or to a city or tea-growing area, I'll bring one or two types just in case, but rely on the tea found there. If camping or traveling to a rural setting, I'll bring more of an array.

My travel lens is tea. I look for a beautiful teahouse or café, but more so, I look for inspiration in dining rooms or kitchen tables, places where I imagine local people enjoy tea. I look for paintings that I'd love to be surrounded by when drinking tea; I look for antique cups and unusual teapots. I look for the velvet couch of my dreams and a sexy dress, the pairing of which would make for a chic tea experience. Having tea as a lens through which you see the world doesn't mean traveling to seek out teahouses or a cup of matcha—it means traveling in a way that centers the tenets of tea culture, such as beauty, simplicity, and relaxation.

Packing Your Own Tea

Whenever we went on a trip anywhere when I was growing up, my mom would always bring her own coffee and French press. I did the same thing when I went on road trips. It's so nice to use the gas station for hot water to pour over your own coffee, versus drinking gas station coffee. For flights, I bring my own tea bags and drink Masha Tea at the gate, waiting to board the plane. It's so easy to get hot water by asking at a coffee shop at the airport.

Similarly, on road trips, good tea and coffee can be difficult to find outside of large cities. Bring tea when taking a local trip with friends. Make tea for everyone first thing in the morning or at the end of a long day. Tea bags are easy to travel with, though it isn't so complicated to bring your own loose tea (along with either a French press or a strainer). If you enjoy making matcha and are visiting family members who don't drink tea, bring your own whisk and matcha setup and make it for yourself and anybody else who wants to try it. Bringing your own tea is about personal comfort—like a child going to her grandparents' house with a beloved stuffed animal; it doesn't mean there aren't other toys that are as good at the house, but yours is there just in case.

A Brief Note about Tea Bags

Loose tea is typically preferable to tea bags because you can choose the preferred amount of tea, are in control of making sure that the leaves are whole and fresh, and there is more of an opportunity to create a moment or ritual. Tea bags can be really useful, though—especially for travel, work, and for making tea for large groups of people. Many tea bags are packaged in single-use plastic envelopes that can't be recycled and the tea bags themselves often contain microplastics. Look for tea in compostable bags; I use these for Masha Tea and now package the bags in refillable tins.

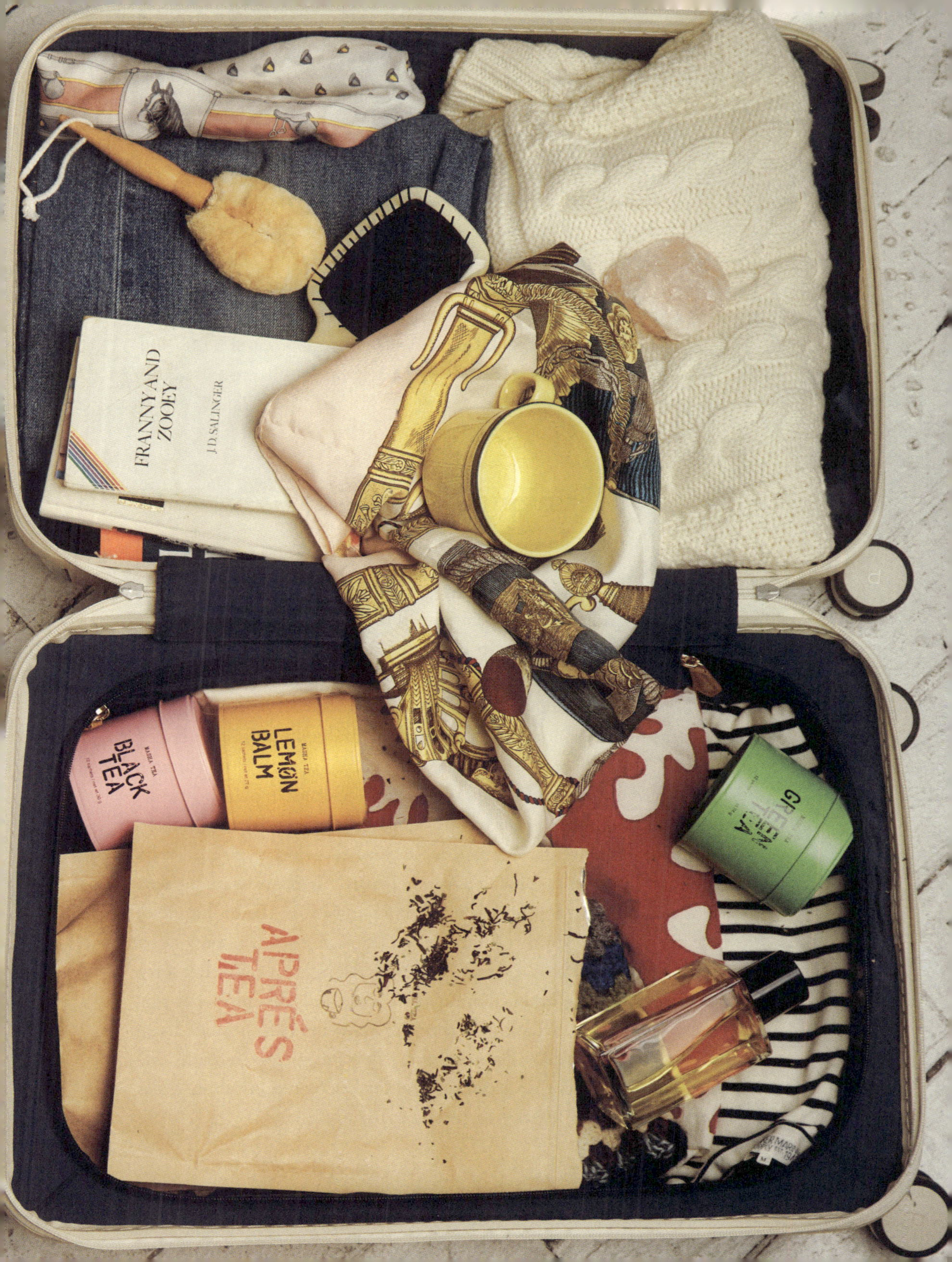
FRANNY AND ZOOEY
J.D. SALINGER
BLACK TEA
LEMON BALM
GREEN TEA
APRÉS TEA

Road Trips

It is simplicity itself to boil water over a campfire and pour it over loose tea in an enamel teapot. In my early twenties, I road-tripped all over the country—the thrill of the open road creates an unparalleled sense of freedom and possibility, especially when you're unrestricted by time and responsibility. It's hard to find fresh food, let alone good tea, in the middle of America, especially when driving on highways. If you're traveling out of a tiny suitcase, wearing the same clothes for weeks, what a touch of home and luxury to have your favorite tea with you.

Drinking Tea in Cities

Visiting organic farms, building relationships with farmers, traveling to rustic corners of the world, and deciding which teas and herbs to source are the best parts of running a tea company. But a close second is visiting the cities where tea customs—whether through ceramics, design, and fashion—are elevated to an art form.

Big cities are exciting amalgamations of culture, tradition, and modernity. Where food, fashion, architecture, and multiculturalism intersect, there is tea. As tea lovers, we have the opportunity to view cities through the unique lens of tea culture. We can look for tea scenes in paintings at art museums, visit gorgeous historical buildings that serve tea in their cafés, picnic with tea in carefully planned parks, and experience teas and ways of drinking tea that are specific to different places. There are so many ways to visit a new city and approaches with which to take in the multitude of possible encounters open to you. Traveling through a tea lens provides a direction and sense of purpose to an itinerary. Along with cafés that serve tea, look for homeware and ceramics shops, spas, and design spaces that incorporate tea and you'll start noticing tea references all around. I will share my experiences with tea in some of my favorite cities to communicate the feeling of their particular tea culture, and to help you think about tea as a way of engaging with any city, anywhere in the world.

New York City

"The girl in the tea shop
Is not so beautiful as she was,
The August has worn against her.
She does not get up the stairs so eagerly;
Yes, she also will turn middle-aged,
And the glow of youth that she spread about us
As she brought us our muffins
Will be spread about us no longer.
She also will turn middle-aged."
— Ezra Pound, *The Tea Shop* (1916)

New York City is my home and so I have the most to say about tea culture here. Going out for tea in New York City doesn't always have to be glamorous. Because coffee house culture permeates the city, drinking tea out in the world is often a mirror of that. A matcha in a paper cup (to go!), a quick hibiscus iced tea out of plastic—such is the pace of the city. Whether we mean to or not, we often accessorize our outfits, meetings, and conversations with the drink we have in hand. The drink reflects our taste in café. When it comes to choosing tea, perhaps it signifies our interest in wellness culture, and it draws attention to our jewelry and well-manicured nails, to how often we're answering the phone that we're holding in our hand, and to our finely glossed lips as we drink out of straws. Drinking tea out isn't usually about the drink in New York. It's about the signifiers. In New York City, tea is best enjoyed at home, whether it be your own home or somebody else's. The coziness of choice in cup and teapot, being able to quiet down and relax and take respite from the world—these moments are more easily obtained in our own controlled environments in New York City, even if those spaces are small apartments. At least they are our small apartments, with our own art on the walls and noise that is relatively predictable.

And yet, I have enjoyed having tea out in this beloved city many times over. I don't write too much about the teahouses themselves—spaces notoriously come and go—though I do love the small Chinese tea shop, Floating

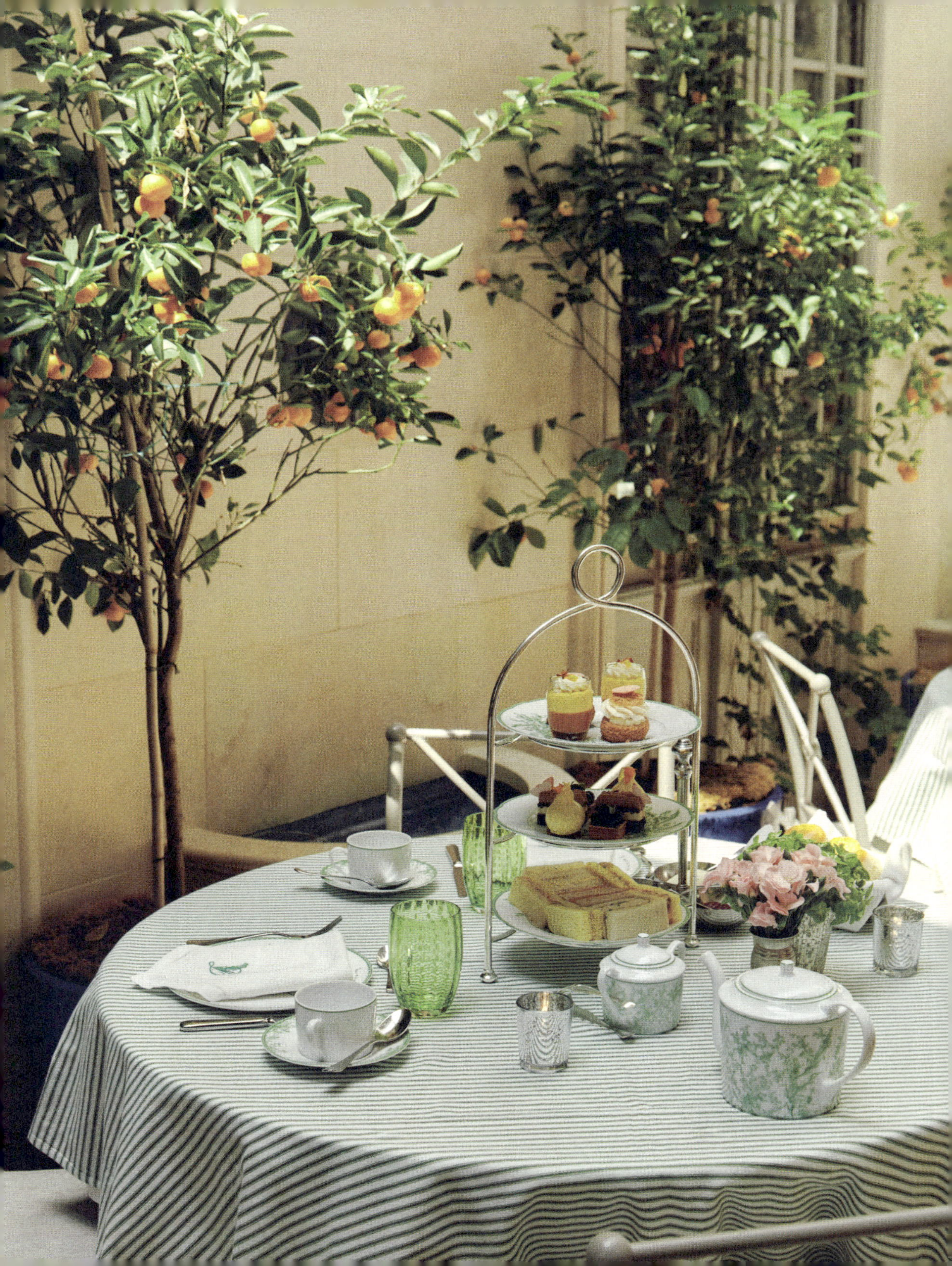

Mountain Tea House, on a second-floor walkup on the Upper West Side, where you must take off your shoes to enter and you can stay as long as you want. I often get pu'erh, a type of tea that I rarely prepare for myself. I love the Taiwanese teahouse in the West Village, Té Company, where I go specifically to drink oolong, another type of tea that I don't often have at home. Perhaps that is one of the points of going out for tea—as with espresso, having it at a café is a superior experience. There are certain types of tea that I rarely include in my home collection, including pu'erhs, oolong, and white tea, and flavored teas such as vanilla. I gravitate toward ordering these teas when I go out. I will almost always choose a vanilla black tea for afternoon tea out (it's a guilty pleasure because there is an element of kitsch and extravagance—it's probably the most expensive way to have tea with sandwiches). I love to try oolongs from Taiwan, aged pu'erhs, and peach-flavored tea when I see it. For me, these are special-treat teas that I don't necessarily want on a regular basis. When ordering tea out, consider what teas you don't have at home and which ones you don't know how to make. If you're not comfortable making matcha at home but love matcha, then it makes sense to go to a great Japanese tea shop instead. If you find yourself coming back for the same tea repeatedly, it might be time to bring it home and incorporate it into your domestic routine.

OUTINGS FOR AFTERNOON TEA

From a practical perspective, afternoon tea in New York can be a place for celebration, a space for a creative business meeting, or a respite for visitors from out of town. On the Upper East Side, not far from Central Park, I love the Lowell Hotel, which has been in the same spot since the 1920s. Their afternoon tea is a collaboration with DIOR, so the teaware, linens, and experience are all curated by the luxury brand, a unique way to enjoy an experiential cosmopolitan fashion outing that doesn't involve shopping.

SAUNA/SPA

One of the secrets of getting through winter in New York is having access to a sauna—and ideally, your sauna serves tea. In a city that is cold, wet, and charmingly inhospitable for many months of the year, it feels incredible to heat up. Exercise does this, as does having tea and soup at home, but nothing truly gets into your bones the way an afternoon in the sauna does. Hotels do this well, including Hotel Chelsea and Shibui Spa in the Greenwich Hotel, but there are also smaller "bathing clubs," infrared saunas, and more local experiences.

MUSEUM CAFÉS AND SHOPS

I first heard of the Noguchi Museum when I moved to New York. The garden, in particular, has since been a place of refuge for me in this city. I wound up curating the tea program at the Noguchi Museum, and Masha Tea was sold there exclusively before the café shuttered during the pandemic. Museum shops invariably have teaware appropriate for the era or style the museum represents. Museum cafés—Cafe Sabarsky at the Neue Gallery, The Modern at the Museum of Modern Art—are among the chicest places to rest for tea after spending an afternoon walking through galleries. When done well, a museum café or restaurant carries the message of the museum into a guest experience—in this case, one around tea.

Los Angeles

With its large Mexican population, L.A. is home to many places to get agua de jamaica, which is sweetened, iced hibiscus tea. There are tea shops in L.A.'s Koreatown serving an array of green tea; invariably mint or black tea served in the homes of the city's large Persian diaspora; and there is afternoon tea served in Beverly Hills hotels. Newer spaces devoted to tea are popping up in the city. While there are some tea shops scattered across Los Angeles, tea culture more typically finds a home in status grocery stores—where you can buy twenty-dollar matcha smoothies—as well as in spas, cute shops, and acupuncture studios, rather than in teahouses themselves.

Pop-wellness culture is about rituals revolving around skincare, meditation, or tea, and making them cute, reproducible, covetable, and attractive. Though there are authentic sources out there, with brands pushing wellness culture, you wind up wondering who is benefiting from a commitment to wellness. Los Angeles is home to many wellness startups focused on superfoods, vitamin powders, efficient meditation, and the embodiment of this culture. One way to experience tea culture in Los Angeles is to lean into the now highly commodified spirit of unapologetic self-care that permeates the city. Angelenos, in the interest of looking good and feeling good (mostly the former), asked, *How does tea benefit me?* And the wellness industry responded. In Los Angeles, matcha is used in smoothies for its antioxidant properties, and herbal teas are incorporated into routines for sleep, beauty, energy, and rest.

From a certain perspective, tea culture exists as a celebration of beauty for the sake of beauty. American notions of beauty, especially for women, center around a perfect notion of the self, of the body, optimally nourished, exercised, rested, and molded into a young, fit form. With wellness culture, which I see so much of in Los Angeles, tea, zero calorie and healthy, fits into that ideal.

Relatively speaking, Los Angeles is a young city, it hasn't been around for thousands of years, and it hasn't even had hundreds of years to establish an infrastructure for tea culture. I think the most fun way to experience tea culture in Los Angeles is through a feel-good wellness lens.

London

"There's a lot to be said for a decent cup of tea,"
a cab driver told me as he drove me to my hotel
in London. "Our country was built on tea."

✣ ✣ ✣

There are spaces all over this city, both grand and unassuming, to drink tea. London is the birthplace of afternoon tea, which is served in some of the city's high-end hotels, such as Claridge's, The Corinthia, and The Ritz, so it's easy to spend afternoons dressed up, having a fancy tea with champagne and pastries. Claridge's, London's quintessential afternoon tea locale, has been serving afternoon tea since the hotel opened in the 1850s.

British afternoon tea begins with a tea menu, with typical black, green, flavored, and herbal choices, and with the option of champagne. The pot of tea comes out with scones, with jam and clotted cream served alongside (clotted cream tastes like a combination of cream and butter). The big drama in England is whether to place the jam or the clotted cream on the scone first.

After the scone course comes tea sandwiches: egg salad, cucumber, smoked salmon, and ham are typical. Then come the pastries. Waiters walk around with carts of dainty cakes, and you get a pastry tray of desserts, sometimes with a theme. The themes can range from seasons to fashion designers. Afternoon tea is an indulgence, but for visitors to the city, it's definitely worth experiencing once during a stay.

Modern-day London is now a hub of international tea traditions and South Asian culture and food. Accordingly, a trip to the city, and an understanding of the city's tea culture, would be incomplete without chai from a traditional Indian or Pakistani kitchen. A fun way to enjoy tea each day, especially if you love chai, is to order it at different Indian and Pakistani establishments throughout the city. The spices used vary by the countries and regions people emigrate from, and restaurants often have house-made regional chai.

Of course, in a city like London, there are teahouses from diasporas the world over and you can find whatever it is you seek. I suggest following up teatime with a walk through one of London's gorgeous parks or gardens.

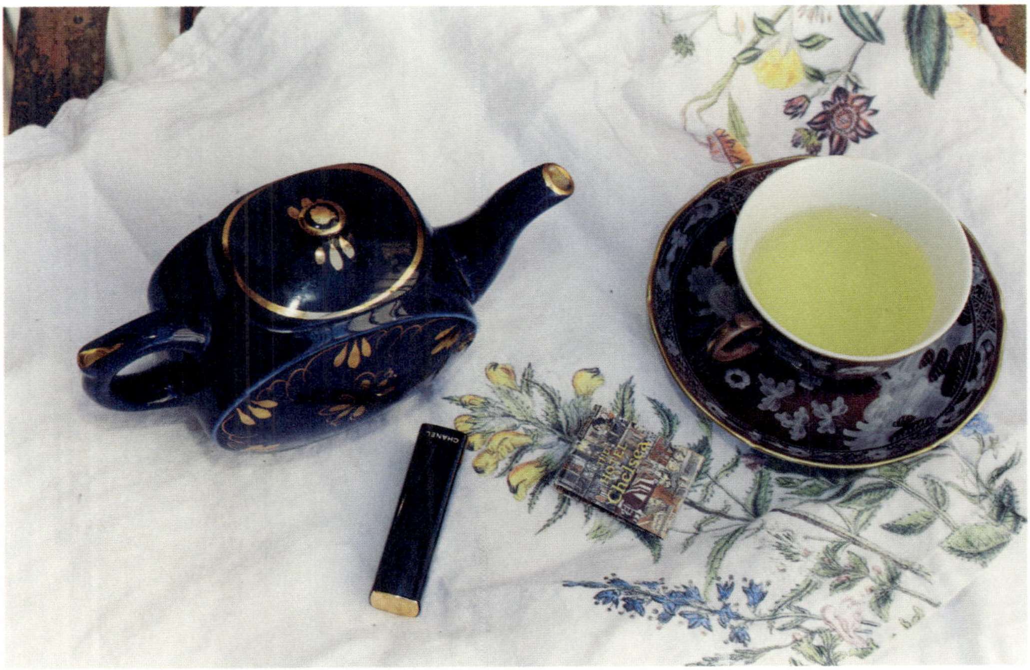
CHANEL
THE HOTEL Chelsea

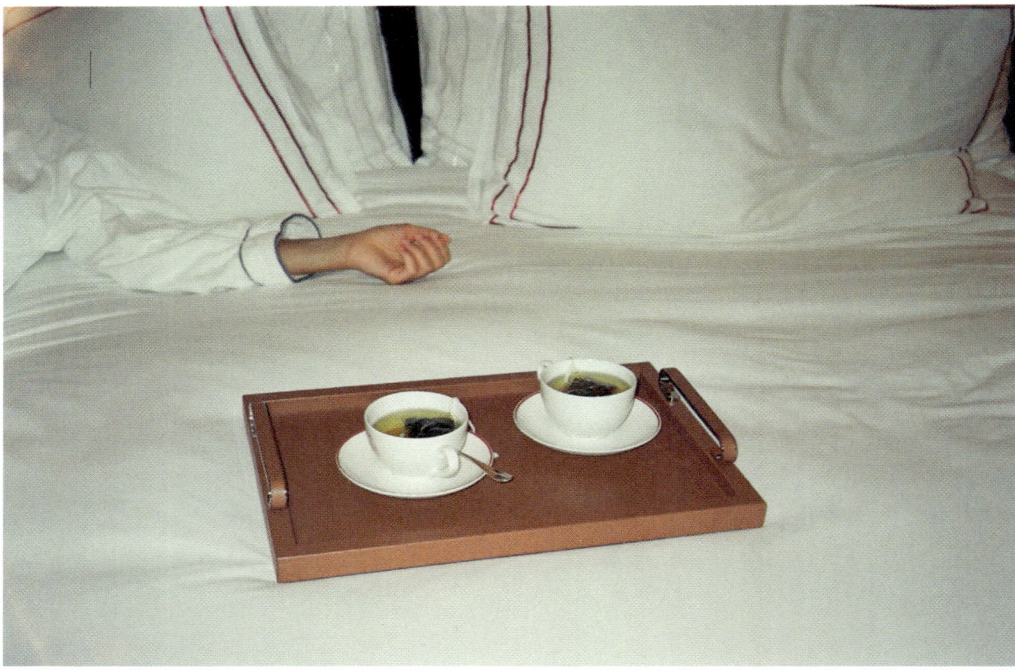

Milan

Given that Italy is a country more famous for its coffee than its tea, I am always pleasantly surprised to see how the experience of tea in the Italian countryside translates seamlessly to the fashion capital of Milan. While the coffee menus at most places are the same (espresso, macchiato, latte), at Milan's tea parlors I found teas from the world over, whether grown in Japan or China, or tisanes from neighboring Germany and from Italy itself.

I also find Milan to offer a different perspective on tea. Whereas in some cities the allure of tea is the beverage or the teahouses, this isn't necessarily the case in Milan—though there are beautiful tea shops. In some ways, Milan is a subtle city. It doesn't have the decadent architecture and design of Rome or Florence, but more of an industrial history and infrastructure. The beauty lies in the intricate details of the building entryways, the houses, the furniture, and in the search for those details. When I focus on tea in culture, I look for the design of a city inspiring its inhabitants to live with tea, and search for specific teas and accoutrements that speak to the city itself. I look for it in movies, books, and paintings about a place. This search makes Milan, at its core a design city, extraordinary.

I first discovered Villa Necchi by watching Tilda Swinton in *I Am Love* (and, later, the villa was featured in *House of Gucci*). Visiting it for the first time in person, amid the meticulously designed rooms, I was delighted to discover the remnants of a family of tea drinkers. There are tea sets in gold, porcelain, and silver; teacups in the paintings on the wall; and perhaps my favorite of all, a plastic red tea set on an unassuming tray in the staff area. In a home-turned-museum, where you can't help but contemplate how a family lived, you can immediately picture them gathering in the garden room, gossiping around cups of tea. Even in *I Am Love,* there's a brief tea scene where Tilda Swinton sits on a couch with her mother-in-law while, in the foreground, one of their maids in a pink dress pours tea from a white porcelain tea set with little pink flowers on it.

This perspective on Milan, of focusing on design and looking for tea culture outside of the teahouse, can be applied to countless cities around the world, though in Milan it takes on a modern, colorful sophistication.

Tokyo

For lovers of tea, there's no place like Japan—from its artful matcha ceremonies to the rolling hills of its tea farms and the spaces in which to drink tea, marked by thoughtful, minimalist design. Since tea originally came to Japan through Zen Buddhism, these spiritual beginnings seem to ripple through to the current day, even in the most metropolitan of places. And with centuries of tea culture in its streets and proximity to some of the most beautiful tea gardens on the planet, Tokyo is one of the world's great tea cities.

Traditional Japanese tea culture revolves around *chadō,* meaning "the way of tea." The ceremony itself is called *chanoyu,* which means "hot water" but is the name for the entire matcha ceremony. Yes, it is a tea ceremony, but it is so much more than that. To become a tea master takes years, so you can extrapolate the difference between that training and the training of a barista, who may learn to make a matcha latte over the course of a couple of days. The structures of a Japanese tea ceremony extend from how to properly walk into a tearoom, to *ikebana,* or the floral arrangements of the room, to *wagashi*-making, which refers to the small, delicious candies that are served with tea. There are masters in *wagashi, ikebana,* and, of course, matcha itself.

As a participant in the tea ceremony, the experience is akin to watching a dance performance. Each move of the hand and body, each sound of the whisk's movement or the kettle pouring, has been calculated to evoke profundity, contemplation, and beauty. Tea ceremony can be experienced in a traditional tearoom, which often has a garden at the entrance, or in less conventional spaces, such as in homes and at hotels.

During a matcha ceremony, the host hands the *chawan* (tea bowl) to the guest with the front (the prettier side) facing the guest. The guest then takes the opportunity to admire the ceramic bowl, the color of the matcha, and the warmth of the bowl before beginning to drink. This aspect of connoisseurship and admiring the collection of tea tools is a key part of the ceremony. The guest can drink the matcha in a few sips, then places the bowl down. Once they're done, the guest rotates the bowl so that the front faces back toward the host, indicating that they're done. The ceremony ends with the host gathering the tea bowls, washing them, and placing them back

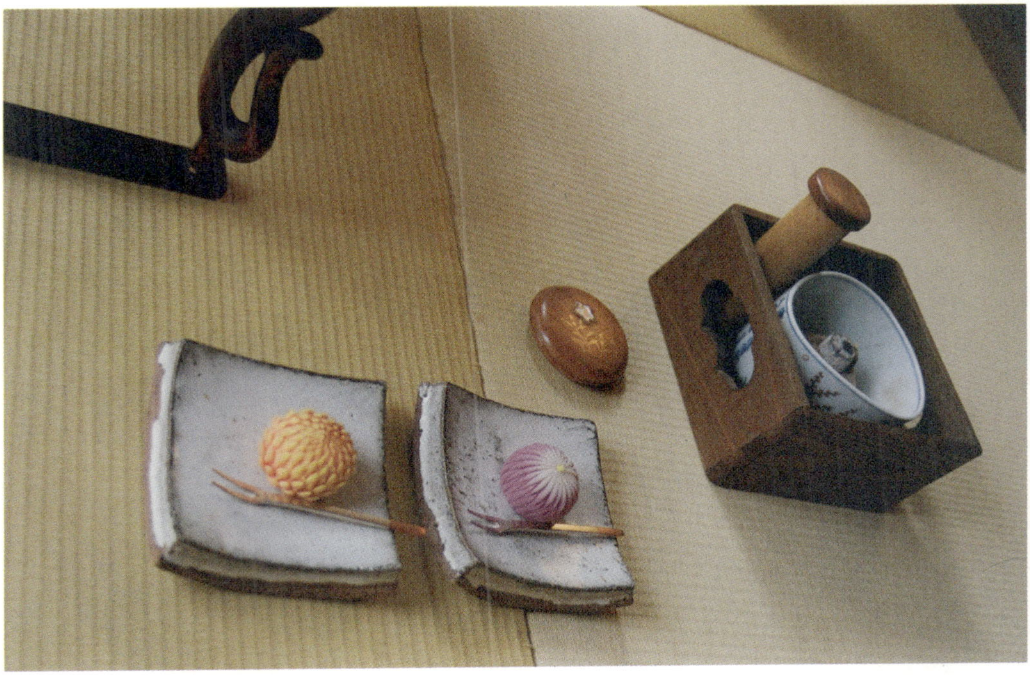

where they are stored, which is often a visible display area. As a guest, a large part of your role is in enjoying and observing the details.

In Tokyo, my favorite cups of tea were in Kagurazaka—a neighborhood referred to both as Little Kyoto and Little Paris for its stone streets, hidden cafés in alleyways, and neighborhood vibe. They were also during a spa day; in the Hoshinoya Hotel, water from a salty hot spring deep underground is brought up to the top floor, where the top of the hotel opens up into the sky like a James Turrell exhibit. In the dressing room you enter and exit the hot spring, and have hot buckwheat tea before and after the soak. Grain teas, like buckwheat, barley, and even toasted rice, are favorite accompaniments before and after a sauna for their savory, nutritious flavor and hydrating mineral profile. *Onsens*, or hot spring baths, are found all over Japan, and no tea lover's visit would be complete without a stop at an onsen town in the Japanese Alps for a stay at a *ryokan*, a traditional inn with tatami mat floors, wood and paper sliding doors, and materials to make tea in each room.

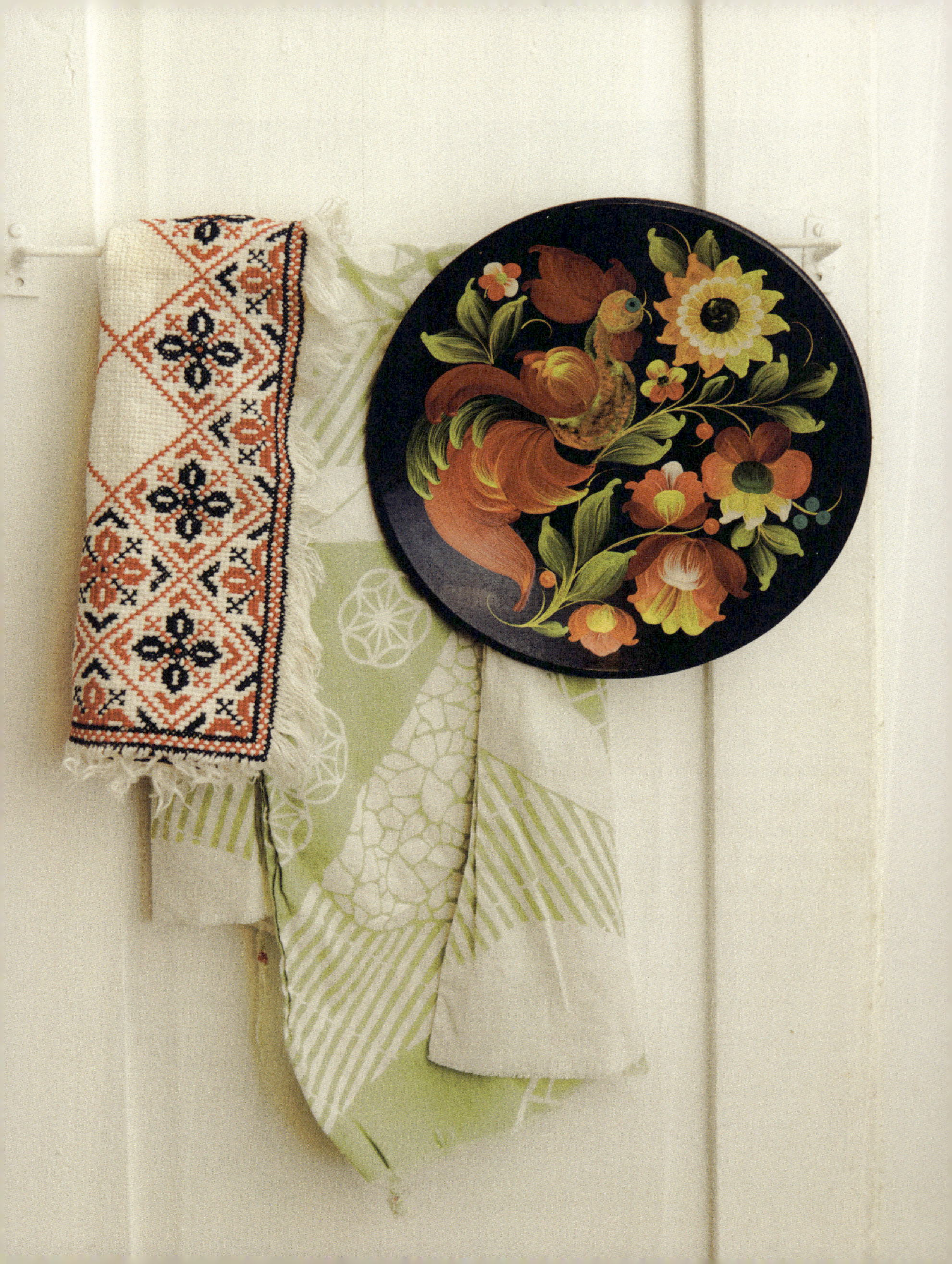

Part 2

Tea at Home

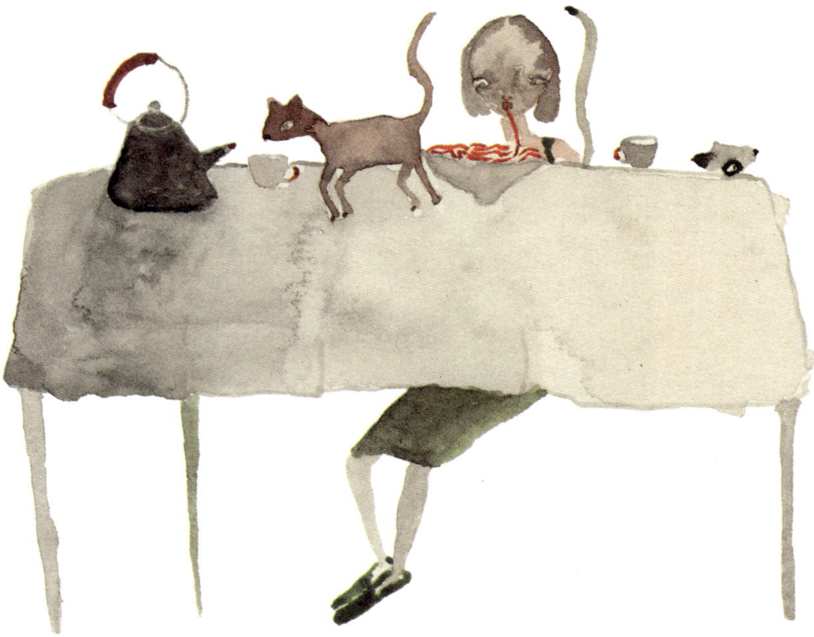

"Style is character."
—Joan Didion, *The White Album* (1979)

– 5 –

Accoutrements

Accoutrements refer to the tools used for a tea service. They include cups and teapots, but also extend to accessories like tea towels, napkins, and silverware. Tea culture is an extension of personal style.

Style has nothing to do with how much money you have and everything to do with confidence, color, and self-expression. Having a sense of personal style makes moving through the world and entertaining more comfortable. Being appropriately dressed for a situation can make you feel confident, at ease, and like you are representing yourself accurately. Your style might express a tendency toward comfort, irony, flirtation. Style is a form of power, a statement, an affirmation of who we are. It makes it more enjoyable to use the tea tools that you buy and have—even if you buy just one item.

If style is taste applied to clothing, then the same sensibilities are naturally used when considering tea service.

My personal style is relaxed, elegant, sexy, and classic. In dress, I gravitate to monochrome colors and prefer natural materials like wool, cotton, and cashmere. Most days, I wear jeans with a T-shirt or sweater. My closet is small, so I tend to buy high-quality pieces that I wear over and over again. I similarly use the same rotating set of porcelain cups and teapots day in and day out. I love to wear dresses and heels on special occasions, and I have glass teapots and pieces that I only bring out for important celebrations. Being detail oriented, I see my hair, nails, skin, and fitness level as an extension of my personal style. I also see what I eat and drink, listen to, and read in the same light. Think about your style and perspective and how it might translate to your choices in tea and teaware.

Style Profiles

Part of having style is knowing yourself and how you like to express yourself. Below are style categories that I've matched with the four elements in Western herbalism, along with some thoughts on manifestations of each.

CLASSIC {fire}

confident, straightforward, powerful, tailored, black, white, and primary colors

The classic tea drinker is moving intentionally through the world, so the cup of tea is a break or a pick-me-up, though their tea collection is carefully considered and of the highest quality. Their teaware collection may include just a handful of favored designers, and their kettle is high-end.

CASUAL {earth}

comfortable, approachable, earth tones

A casual tea drinker might choose teas that they know benefit their health and body. Their teaware collection feels handmade, with organic shapes in brown hues. Their clothes are durable and made from natural materials. For tea on the go, they have a well-loved thermos that goes everywhere with them.

FORMAL {air}

exclusive, romantic, bejeweled

A formal tea drinker's tea of choice is expensive, considered, and difficult to pronounce. They have carefully chosen the proper tools for their meticulously crafted tea times and they may serve a multicourse meal with a tea pairing, or carefully made delicate desserts. They commit to rituals, whether it be tea time, meditation, exercise, or a skincare routine.

ECLECTIC {water}

drawn to color, mismatched, fluid, with a collector's mindset

When having tea, an eclectic tea drinker would prefer to sit on a comfortable floor pillow, trying a new tea blend in a cup from their extensive travel collection. Their tea cabinet is huge—some of the pieces many years old. They have colorful tea towels and interesting rugs and curtains.

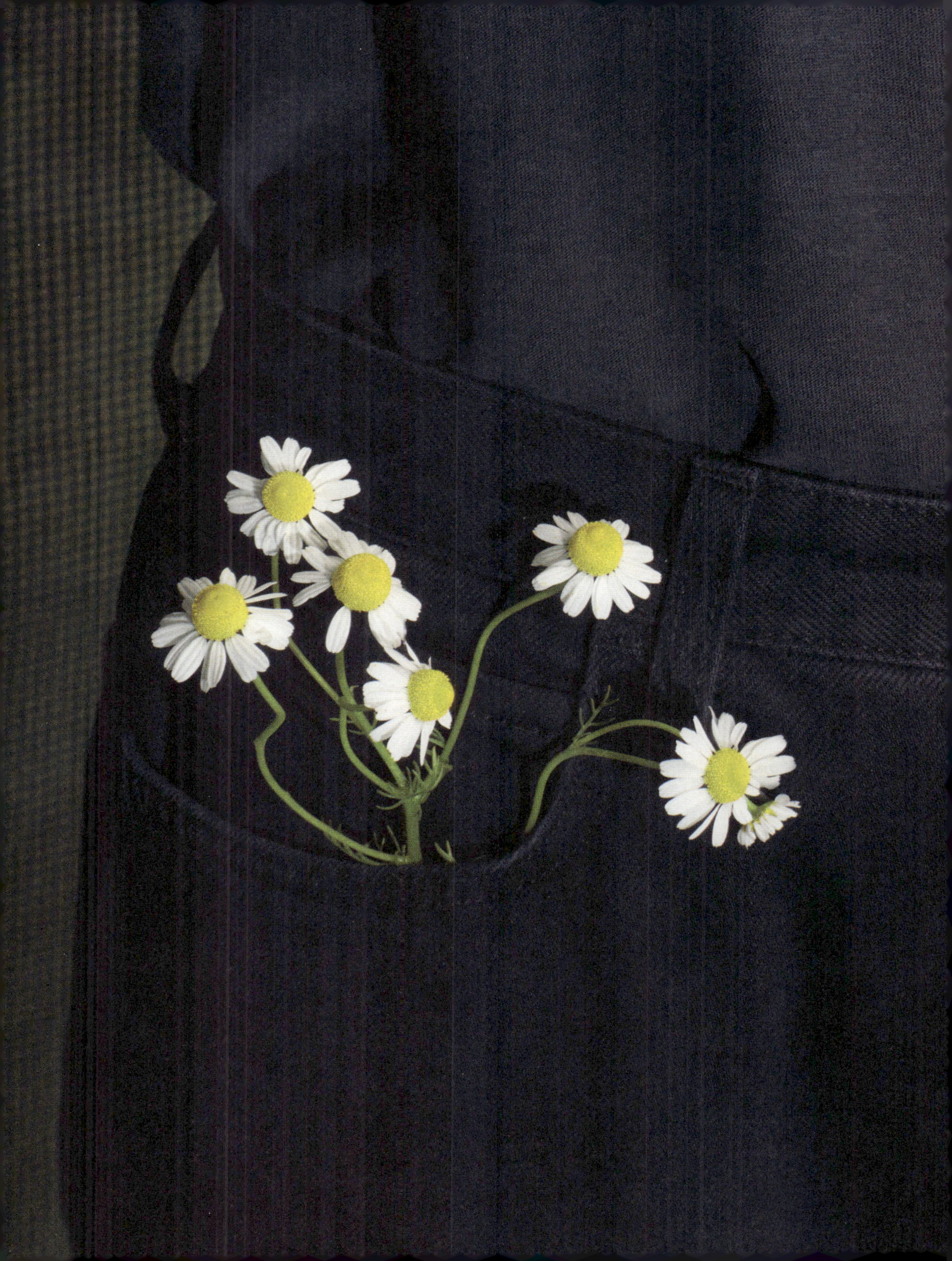

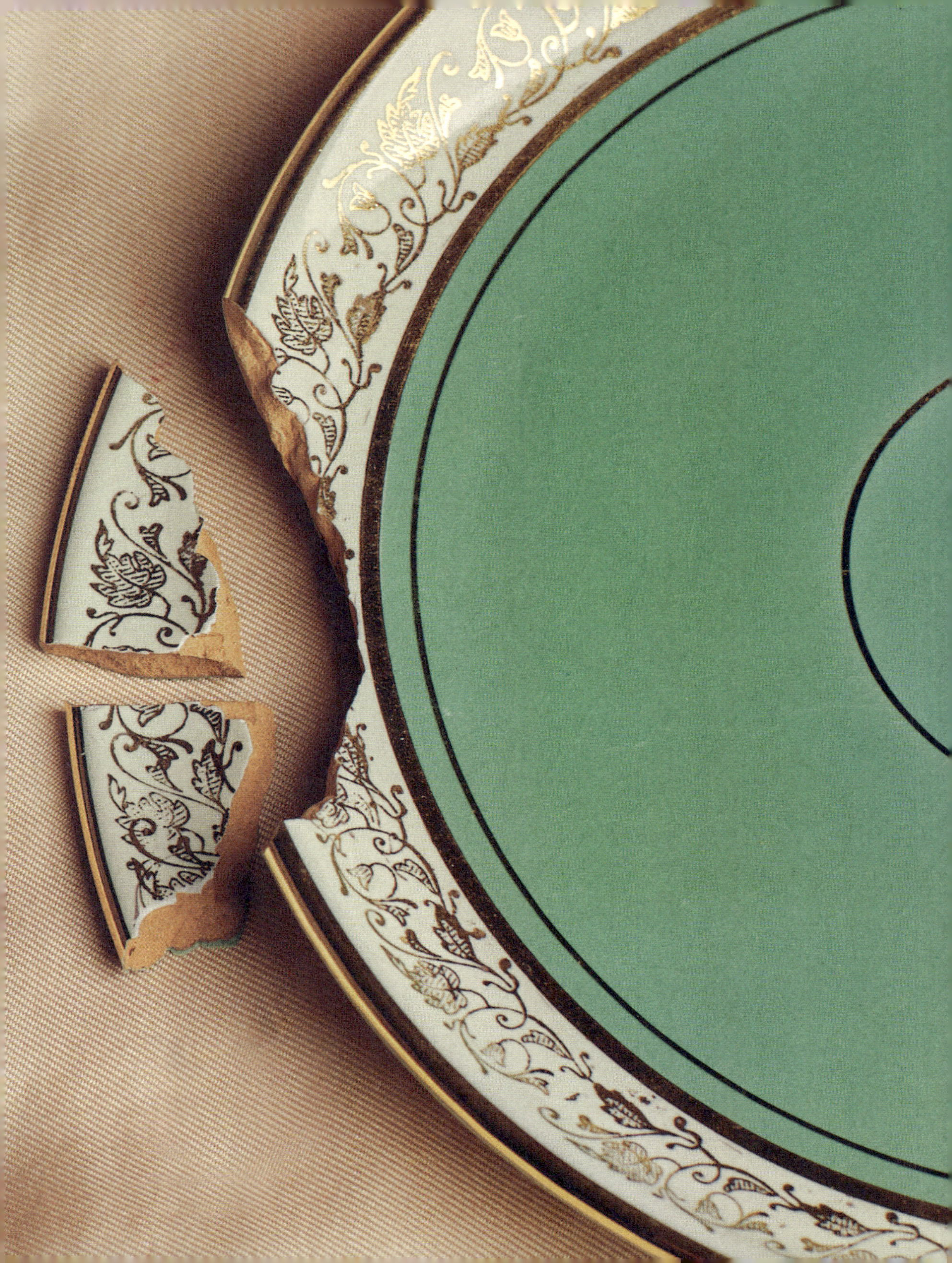

Materials

The choice of material used for teaware greatly impacts the experience of having tea. You can choose materials based on utility, interior design considerations, and your attachment to the objects themselves. When choosing materials for serving tea, think about how well the material conducts heat, how long the tea will stay hot, and whether you would burn your hand or mouth by touching it. Then think about how looking at it or touching it would make you feel—and maybe learn the backstory of the material.

Clay

Clay was traditionally harvested near bodies of water and then molded to make pots or teaware. Today, clay manufacturers produce clay from dry raw materials, making specific clays reproducible for market. After being molded into a cup, bowl, or teapot, clay is glazed and then heated in a kiln to make the shape hold, and for it to be food safe. There's a lot of room for personal expression with clay—of course, it's reflective of the artist making it, but also the taste and sensibilities of the person choosing which piece to bring home. When it comes to clay and personal style, homemade, handbuilt ceramics may reflect a love for artistry and craft. Collecting ceramics during travel creates an eclectic mix and a simple way to integrate travel experiences into your lifestyle.

STONEWARE

Stoneware and porcelain are two types of clay used in food-safe materials. There are other types of clay, like earthenware, which are more typically used for things like tile and terracotta. Stoneware is usually heavier, made from denser material, and has an earthy color when fired. Porcelain, which is fired at higher temperatures than stoneware, is more delicate, dries a bright white color after firing, and is more difficult to work with because it dries quickly. Most designer teaware is made from porcelain.

Some of my most prized possessions are the many tea sets that my grandparents brought with them when they immigrated to New York. I recently found that they mostly come from the same porcelain factory in Ukraine.

Cast Iron

I didn't consider using cast iron for tea until I found a vintage Japanese teapot in a thrift store in Wyoming. Cast iron holds heat in and so keeps tea hot for a long time. Cast-iron kettles can be heated on the stovetop, however, just like cast-iron pans, they get extremely hot so you need to use an oven mitt or pot holder when handling. This doesn't happen with cast-iron teapots because the handle never gets an opportunity to heat up in that way. I think of cast iron as masculine and moody. Most cast-iron teaware is black, making it fitting for a Gothic-inspired setting. Because cast iron keeps tea quite hot, I like to make black tea in it, which is ideal at higher temperatures, versus more delicate green or white teas.

Glass

Glass for teaware feels pretty and young. Similar to ceramics, hand-blown glass leaves a lot of space for creativity and individuality in shape and color. It's ultimately not a great material for hot tea because it loses heat so quickly. I have a glass teapot that also has a glass filter on the inside, which was a poor design for a filter as it gets leaves stuck in it and needs to be cleaned. I have a small glass teapot that has a metal spiral that serves as the filter. This is much better and hasn't broken because, though the glass is delicate, the part that needs to be diligently cleaned is a different material. The best glass pieces are small, because you drink the tea quickly, before it has the chance to cool. With clear glass, you can see the color of the tea, which is why I like to use glass for hibiscus tea, which is bright red, and for hōjicha, which is a deep honey color. I have a set of thick Korean glass teacups, which are quite small and so work for drinking hot tea. The thickness prevents the glass from getting too hot to the touch, and the size makes the tea cool down quickly.

I consider glass fitting for adding femininity to a table, for pairing well with light colors, and also for overlapping between teaware and florals. The same cups of Murano glass, which are often bright and colorful, can be used both as cups for iced tea and as vases for small bouquets of flowers. How lovely for a table setting.

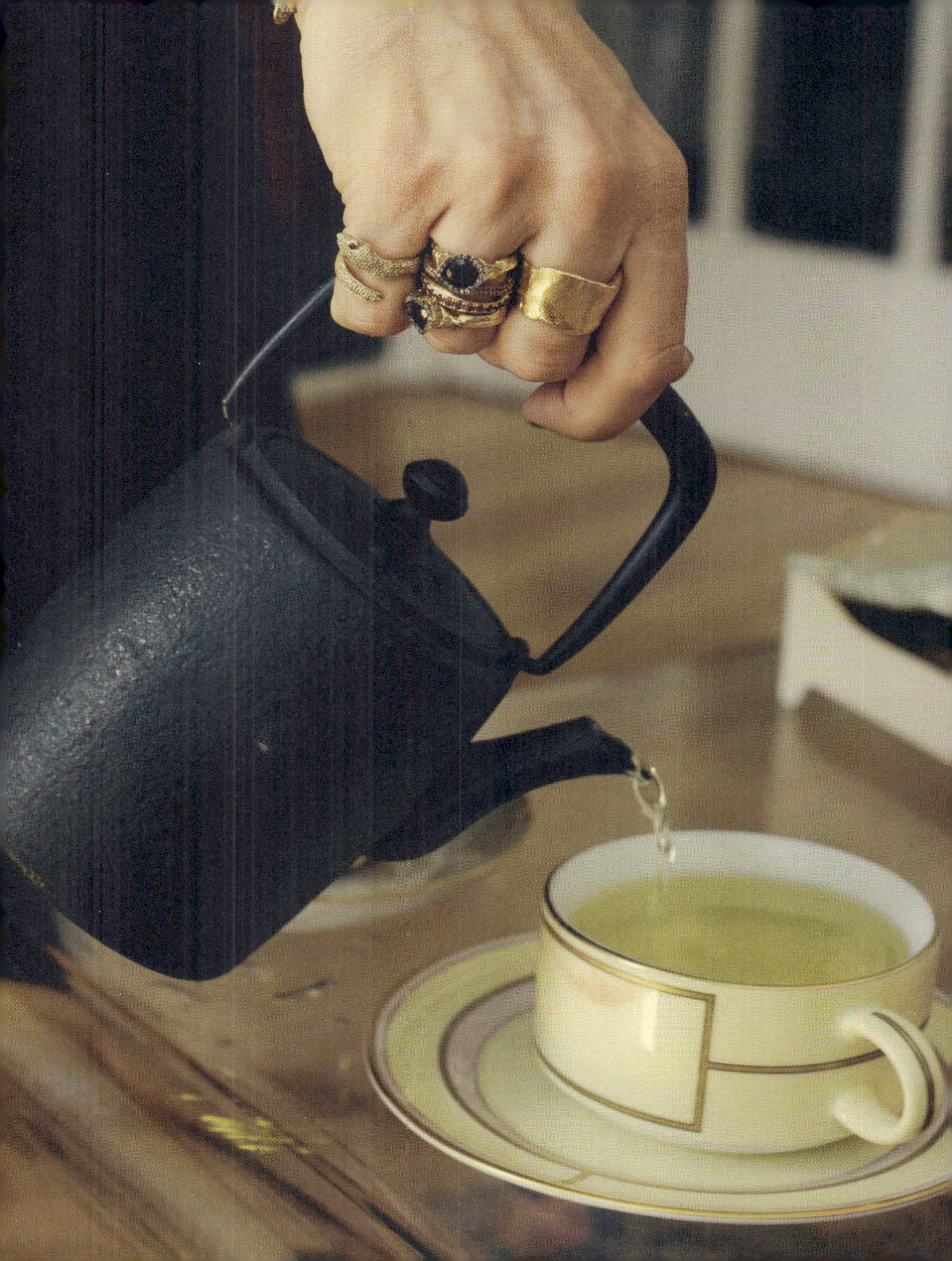

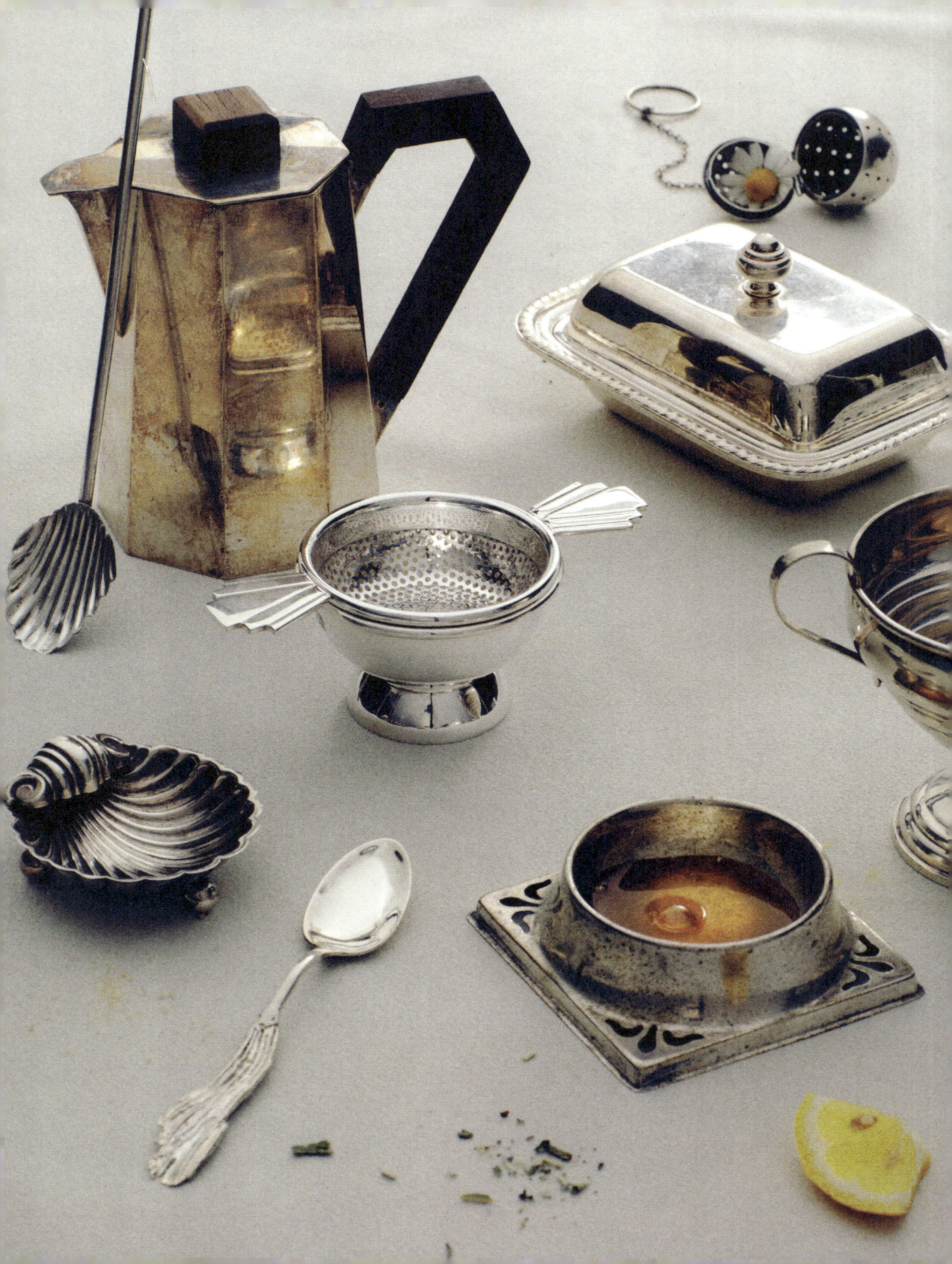

Silver

Sterling silver teaware is much more expensive and rare than silver plated, the latter typically covering brass or a different metal beneath it. Silver, or silver-plated, teapots might reflect a more formal tea drinker—someone who views their teaware as an extension of their jewelry collection. Silver might be used for special occasions, so bringing out the silver could also signify a celebration like a holiday or birthday party.

Enamel

Enamel is made from a mix of porcelain and metal, which makes it lightweight but also makes it stay hot to the touch. Porcelain enamel (also called vitreous enamel) is different than porcelain clay. The latter is typically kaolin clay, whereas porcelain enamel is a powdered glass dipped, typically in steel, for teaware. Enamel can also be dipped in stone, pottery, glass, and metal. Someone who enjoys camping and hiking might collect enamel teaware because its lightweight nature makes it ideal for preparing tea outdoors. It is associated with a more casual style.

Bamboo

Where it's not indigenous, bamboo is an invasive species that grows rapidly and often takes over forests. A bamboo forest is one single colony connected by a rhizome structure beneath. It is a grass rather than a tree, a quality that you can see in the way that it sways.

Matcha whisks and spoons are traditionally made from bamboo, with high-quality ones being made from a single piece. Other uses of bamboo in a tea context include bamboo handles on cups and teapots.

When I was growing up in New Jersey, there was a bamboo forest a ten-minute drive from my house. I loved watching the bamboo move in the wind. My most recent visit to a bamboo forest was in Japan, on a visit to one of the tea farms in Shizuoka, where I source some of my tea. The farm is on mountainsides beside national forest land and there were patches of bamboo growing there, to the dismay of the farmers.

Gold

When it comes to teaware, gold acts as more of an accessory than a main ingredient. The material is somewhat impractical, as it's quite soft. Instead, gold tableware is usually stainless steel, made mostly of chromium and nickel, plated with gold. For this reason, gold tableware can look tacky and inexpensive. Where gold is so alluring in teaware is in the subtle details of teacups and plates.

There are several processes for applying gold to ceramics, including gold leaf (gilding) and paintbrushing (gold luster), with the gold typically being applied before a final porcelain firing. The gold technique in pottery that is most famous, and perhaps most intriguing, is kintsugi.

KINTSUGI

"When the bowl broke, that was my heart.
Laughter fell out."
—Beatrice Wood,
I Shock Myself: The Autobiography of Beatrice Wood (1988)

Kintsugi, also known as *kintsukuroi,* translated to golden joinery and golden repair respectively, is a Japanese art form dedicated to repairing broken ceramics using gold powder and the resin of Urushi trees. In Japan, Urushi has been used for over nine thousand years, since the Jōmon period, to repair vessels. Kintsugi dates back to the early Edo period in Japan, about four hundred years ago, during the birth of the Japanese tea ceremony. At that time, when tea ceremony was a culture specific to the wealthy, the tea vessels were extremely valuable and one-of-a-kind, leading to a desire to preserve and repair them when broken. The philosophy behind kintsugi involves turning something broken and imperfect into something beautiful.

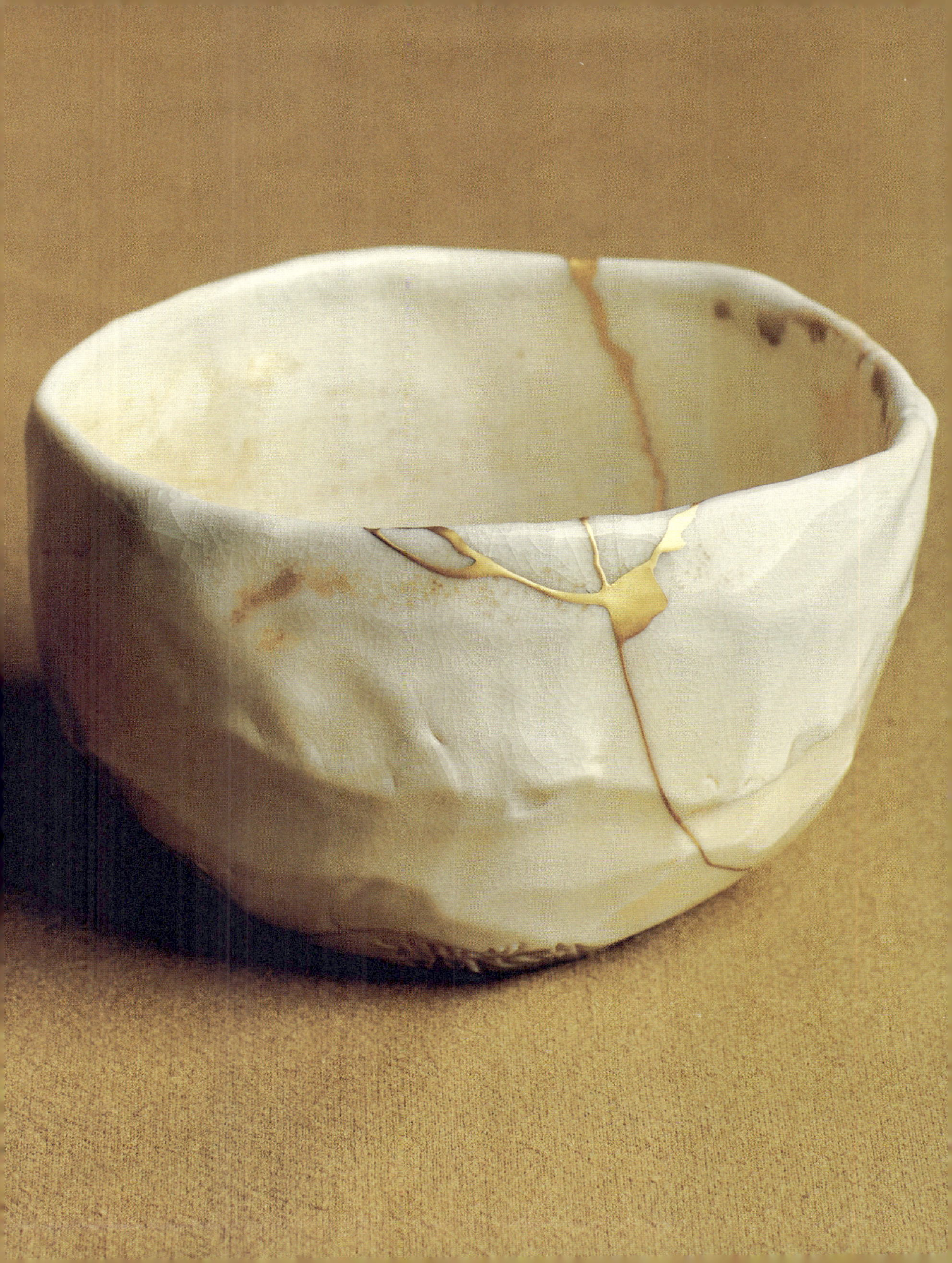

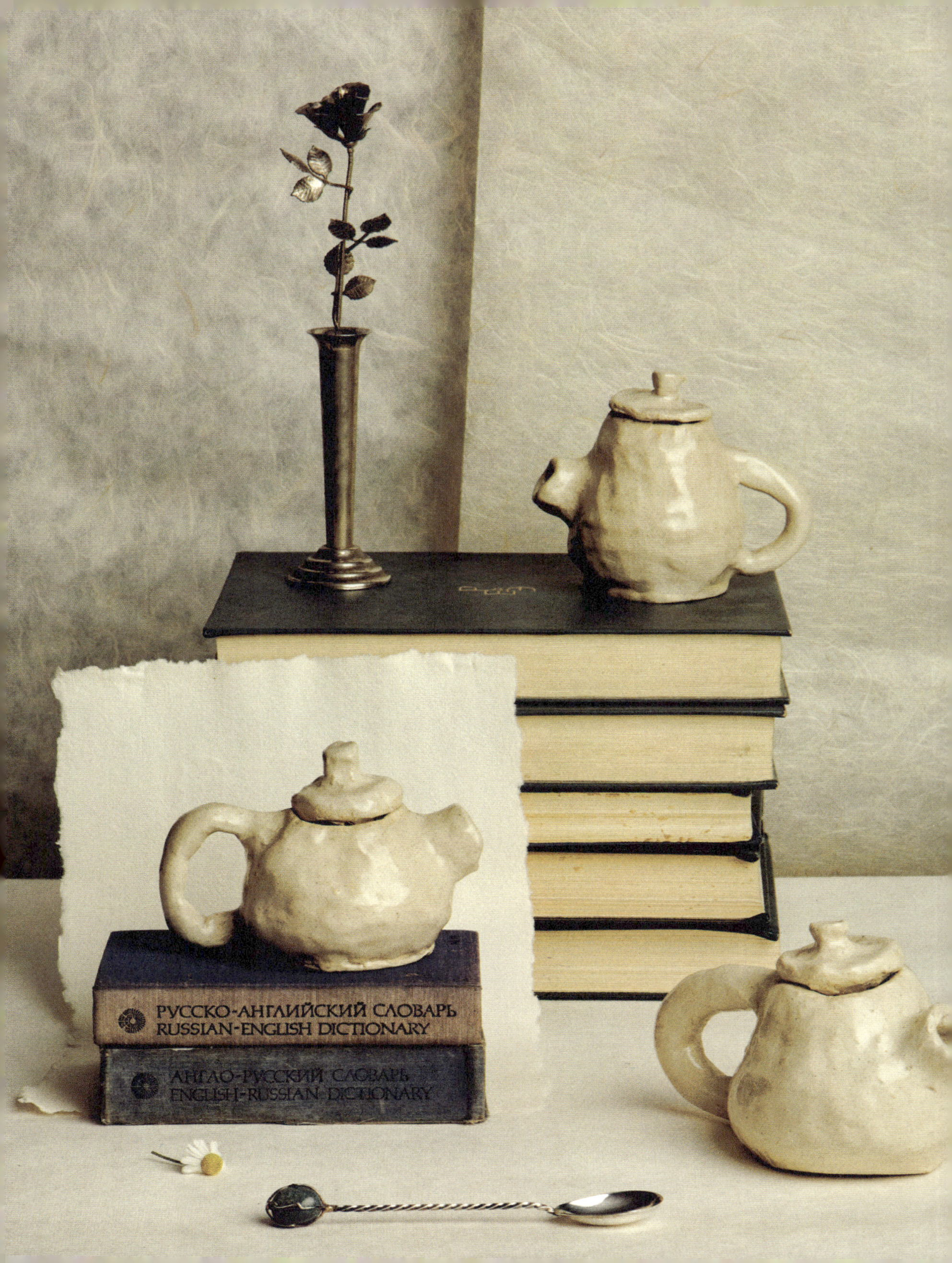
РУССКО-АНГЛИЙСКИЙ СЛОВАРЬ
RUSSIAN-ENGLISH DICTIONARY
АНГЛО-РУССКИЙ СЛОВАРЬ
ENGLISH-RUSSIAN DICTIONARY

Tools

You only need a saucepan, water, herbs, and a stovetop to make tea. But a well-equipped tea drinker also owns materials like strainers and temperature-controlled kettles. Consider your needs. Ultimately, making tea should be simple and enjoyable.

For those whose personal style is clean and consistent, there is much room for precision in tea culture. Weight of tea leaves, temperature of water, and brewing time are key. For those with a more intuitive style, you might opt to eyeball tea in a spoon versus buying a kitchen scale, and you might decide that tea is brewed enough based on its color rather than its temperature. Either approach can be appropriate.

By understanding the tools at your disposal when it comes to making tea, you can choose which ones to incorporate into your daily life, which ones to have on hand for special occasions, and which to either forgo or consider as a gift for somebody who enjoys tea.

There are classic floral patterns that tie pieces to England, or shapes that are clearly Japanese, all potentially made from the same or a similar material: clay. There are those cultural gestures in clay, emblematic of a place or time. With handmade pieces, each one is slightly different from its neighbor, in form and color. These pieces, whether stoneware or porcelain, are made on a potter's wheel or hand-built in a potter's studio.

For a home collection, consider getting a matching tea set, or choosing a couple of colors and collecting pieces in that colorway for a cohesive set. Or embrace having mismatched ceramics. It's fun to have a mix of sizes, shapes, and colors and allow guests to choose their own.

A favorite of mine is a mismatched porcelain collection of cups and saucers made in West Germany and England, sourced in the South of France. I received this as a gift: cups with reds, royal blue, periwinkle, bright sunflowers in similar but not identical proportions. They bring me so much joy—deciding which one to use every day, guessing which friends will drink out of which one, having tea with my husband and daughter, and allowing my young daughter to learn how to drink tea out of something so special, realizing it's better that she uses it and it breaks than it doesn't get used at all.

Teapots

A teapot can be plump, tall, adorable, stately, functional, nice-looking but poorly designed, tiny, enormous, the perfect size for two, the right size for six, kind of funny looking, intimidating, or perfect for a country home. I have many. You too can have a teapot collection. Or you can have just one or two teapots: one for everyday use and another for special occasions. Perhaps the latter is larger in size so you can make tea for two or for a party. Selecting a teapot is something of a practical affair as well: I've had several that spill all over the place when pouring, and that's not ideal, but teapot selection should also come from the heart. There are so many beautiful pieces out there and you should truly love your choice.

Kettles

ELECTRIC: Differences with electric kettles are mostly aesthetic. Gooseneck models are typically used for pour-over coffee and are not really necessary for tea, unless you enjoy the shape. Many brands make them across price points. One useful feature of some electric kettles is the ability to control temperature. So, if you want to brew a gentle white tea at 185°F, for example, you could do that and you could opt to keep the kettle heating at that temperature. This style of electric kettle is the simplest way to measure temperature for tea at home.

STOVETOP: Stovetop kettles should have a cover over the spout so you know when the tea has boiled. I once had a stovetop kettle with a gooseneck that would spurt water all over the place when it boiled over, never making any noise or giving any indication that the water was ready. A stovetop kettle should be functional and attractive, and, because it has a permanent home on the stove, is a way to make an intentional style choice through color and form in the kitchen.

Teacups

When it comes to selecting teacups, consider size, appearance, and material. Of course, it's lovely if you have cups that match the teapot, but I like to use different cups for specific occasions. My "Books you don't need in a place you can't find" diner-style mug (heavy ceramic) from a bookstore in Massachusetts is the one I use in the mornings for a cup of black tea with milk. I use tiny Japanese teacups for sharing several brews of a small pot of tea with a friend. I use a matching set when I have many people over. I use my grandmother's set when my sister visits, and I use thick Korean glass teacups when my husband and I are drinking tea together. Teacups are a fine item to collect. You can pick up different styles on your travels and suit them to any need.

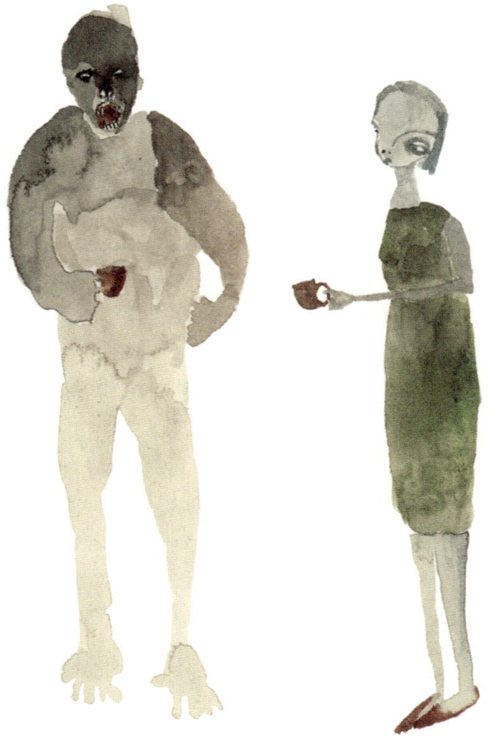

Tea-Leaf Infusers

Infusers serve the dual purpose of brewing tea leaves and then straining them. Having an infuser is essential for brewing loose tea as a way to seamlessly separate the leaves from the water. Options exist for truly gorgeous infusers, or for teapots with infusers built into them. In a bind, creativity will take you far, and you can always use a simple kitchen strainer.

SINGLE-PORTION INFUSERS: After infusing, loose tea should be strained before drinking. If making tea in one-cup potions, use bamboo, ceramic, or metal mesh strainers that fit over the cup's opening. Functionally, I never recommend using the ball-style infuser, because they are awkward to get tea into and ultimately make a mess, so use only for aesthetic purposes. Instead, opt for infusers that you can set on top of a cup.

MULTI-PORTION INFUSERS: Some teapots come with wire-mesh strainers in the center that you portion the tea leaves directly into. Some ceramic teapots come with little holes built into the design to catch the tea leaves before they are poured out into a cup. If your teapot does not have either of these options, pour the tea over a fine-mesh strainer into the cups.

For any of these methods, have a small dish nearby to place the infuser onto, as one does with tea bags.

GAIWAN: This is a Chinese style of brewing tea. It is also the name of the little bowl with lid that you use to make it. You pour with one hand and use the lid to prevent the tea leaves from being poured into the cup.

FRENCH PRESS: Technically these are used to make coffee, though a French press is a really simple way to brew tea, especially tea that has been cut and sifted into small pieces, which happens more often with herbal blends. It might not be the correct or most attractive way to brew tea, but it works. If you drink both tea and coffee, I would suggest having separate French presses for each, as the coffee smell can never be fully washed out of a French press.

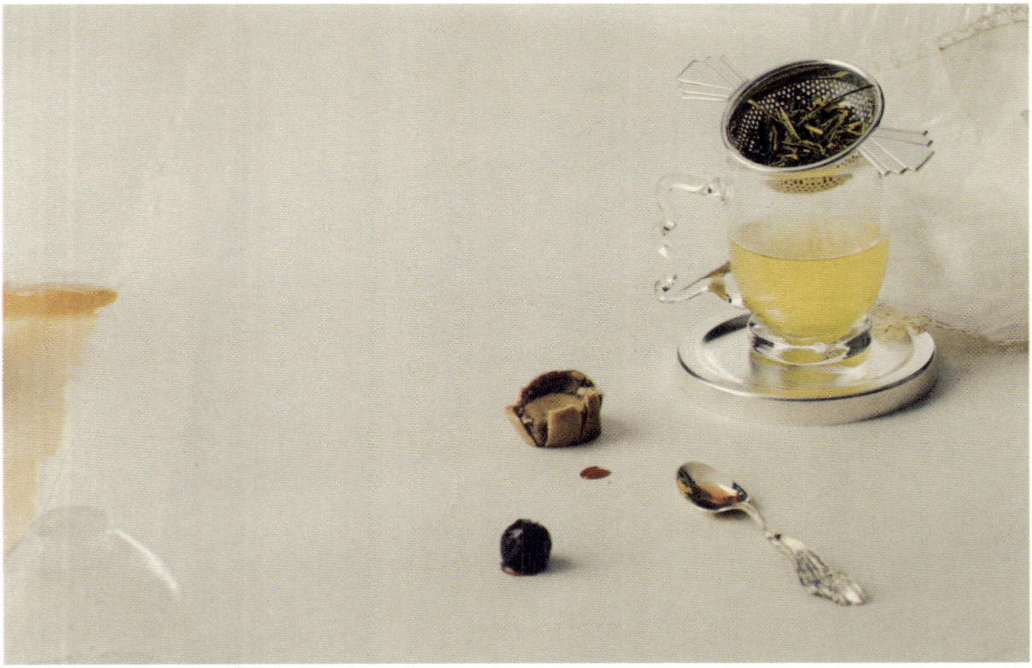

Tea Storage

Tea doesn't expire, but it does lose freshness and potency, especially when exposed to oxygen. If stored in the dark, away from sunlight, in a moisture-free and airtight container, tea won't mold. It stays safe to drink for years, though it does lose flavor and efficacy. Leaves, roots, and flowers maintain their medicinal properties for about a year. Barks and seeds maintain their medicinal properties for two to three years. If you don't drink a lot of tea, metal tins are your best option. Since I drink a lot of tea, I often use glass tea-storage jars. These containers are really lovely for display purposes and are a great way to keep tea, if you go through it quickly. For Masha Tea, we sell loose teas in compostable bags for sustainability reasons, with the understanding that people go through the bags quickly. Matcha is best stored in the fridge because the powder has more surface area exposed to oxygen than a full leaf, so it loses freshness faster.

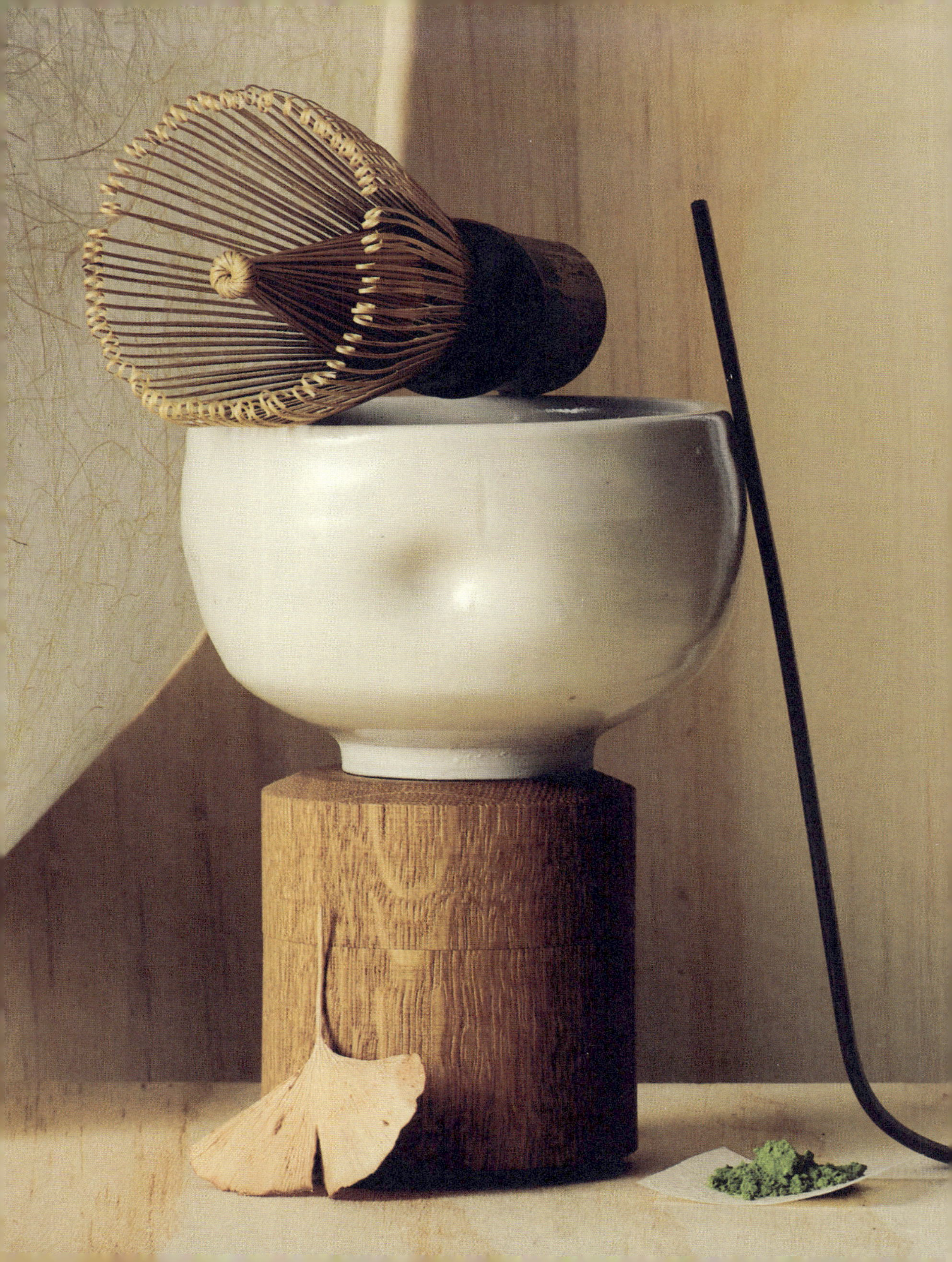

Matcha Tools

When making matcha, you need a whisk, a spoon, and a tea bowl. A second bowl is often needed into which to pour the hot water so that it cools before it is poured over the matcha, though if you have a temperature-controlled kettle, you can set it to about 160°F and then not worry about the water cooling down on its own. A small fine-mesh strainer is also recommended to sift the matcha from its tin to the cup.

Additional Tools

For people who enjoy precision in tea-making, you can use a scale, thermometer, and timer. A simple baking scale that measures in grams will do. Most servings of tea, including matcha, are about 3 grams per cup. For temperature, you'll want a programmable kettle that allows you to brew to a specific temperature. This is more accurate and seamless than an instant-read thermometer. To be sure your tea isn't over or under brewed, you'll need a timer. Under brewed tea will taste too watery, without enough flavor coming through, and over brewed tea tends to turn bitter.

Tea Spaces

When it comes to the spaces in which we drink tea, outside of Japanese teahouses, British tearooms, and other formal places, consider creating your own special corners and spaces for tea in the home. Do you have room for floor pillows, is there a seat near a sunny window, do you have a favorite chair? Furniture is an extension of personal style, and it's an extension of the concept of accoutrement.

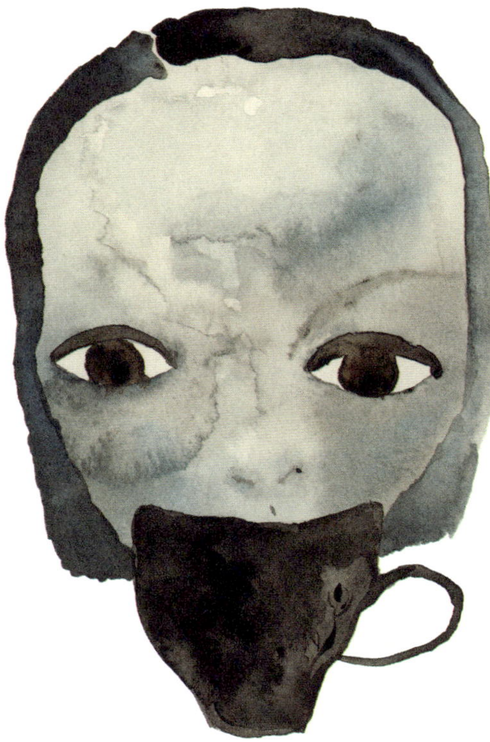

"The best mountain water drips down from stalactites or flows unhurriedly through gravel ponds . . . When boiling water begins to produce bubbles like fishes' eyes and there is some sound, that is the first boil; when the edge froths are like a string of pearls, that is the second boil. When it seethes in waves, that is the third boil. Boiling beyond this stage makes the water stale and unsuitable for drinking."

—Lu Yu, *The Classic of Tea* (780 AD)

– 6 –

Making Tea

Anyone can make an excellent cup of tea. To do so, you'll need confidence, a willingness to experiment, and great ingredients. Through learning to make a simple cup of hot tea, iced tea, matcha, or tea ice pops (in summer), you can begin to incorporate tea into your daily life. The recipes in this chapter can be applied to many different kinds of teas and herbs. Once you use the recipes to the point of understanding how they work, you will be able to make tea without a reference. The more you read about, smell, pick, taste, and drink herbs, the deeper your relationship with them becomes. By learning to trust your own taste, you develop intuition. The goal is to develop your intuition to the point where you don't need a recipe and know how to approach different plants for tea making.

On the packaging for the Masha Tea matcha, it reads, "half a teaspoon per cup of water or make intuitively." It has been that way for years, and I didn't think much of it until a friend pointed out recently how emblematic that instruction is of my approach. My grandmother's recipes were always that way, too. She would say things like use "enough" flour for a recipe or "a handful" of raisins. We are born with instinct, but intuition is something that we all subconsciously develop and hone over time. To develop intuition about how to make tea, you'll incorporate what you've learned about sourcing great tea and using fresh water, and apply the basic recipes that follow.

Since tea is mostly water, the flavor and quality of your water will affect the flavor and quality of the tea, which is why I prefer to use filtered or spring water. One main flavor consideration with tap water is chlorine, which is in all tap water for disinfection purposes. Some people are quite sensitive to this taste. The taste usually dissipates if you leave water out on the counter for three or four hours, or better yet, use a water filter.

Black Tea

Serves 1

This recipe is for a simple cup of tea, something that everybody can easily make. Being able to make a great cup of hot tea will improve your life. With the recipe here and those that follow, double them, triple them, extrapolate the ratios as needed based on whether you're making tea for yourself, for two, or for a group. I grew up drinking over-brewed black tea, and this is still how I like it. I sometimes drink black tea with honey and milk or lemon, but usually just have it black. The longer you brew black tea, the more tannic it becomes. Tannins impart astringency, which is a slightly drying feeling in the mouth and a bitter flavor.

Teapot

Electric kettle with temperature setting (optional)

Fine-mesh tea strainer

Teacup

✢ ✢ ✢

1 teaspoon (3 g) loose black tea leaves, such Darjeeling, Assam, Earl Grey, or Lapsang souchong

1 cup (240 ml) water, preferably filtered

Place tea in teapot. Heat the water to 190 to 212°F (boiling) [88 to 100°C]. Pour the boiling water over the tea and steep for 3 to 5 minutes, depending on strength preference. Strain into a teacup.

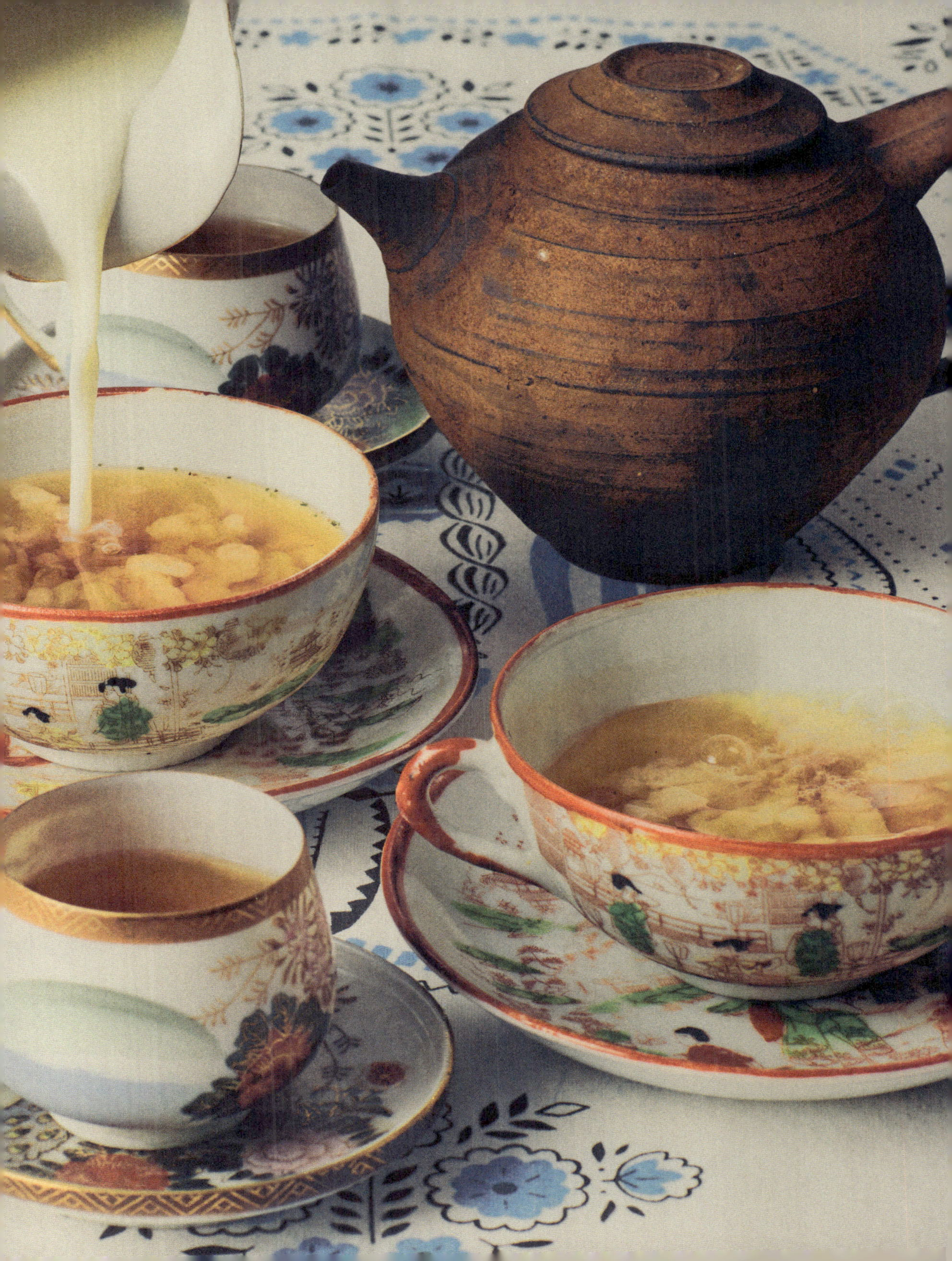

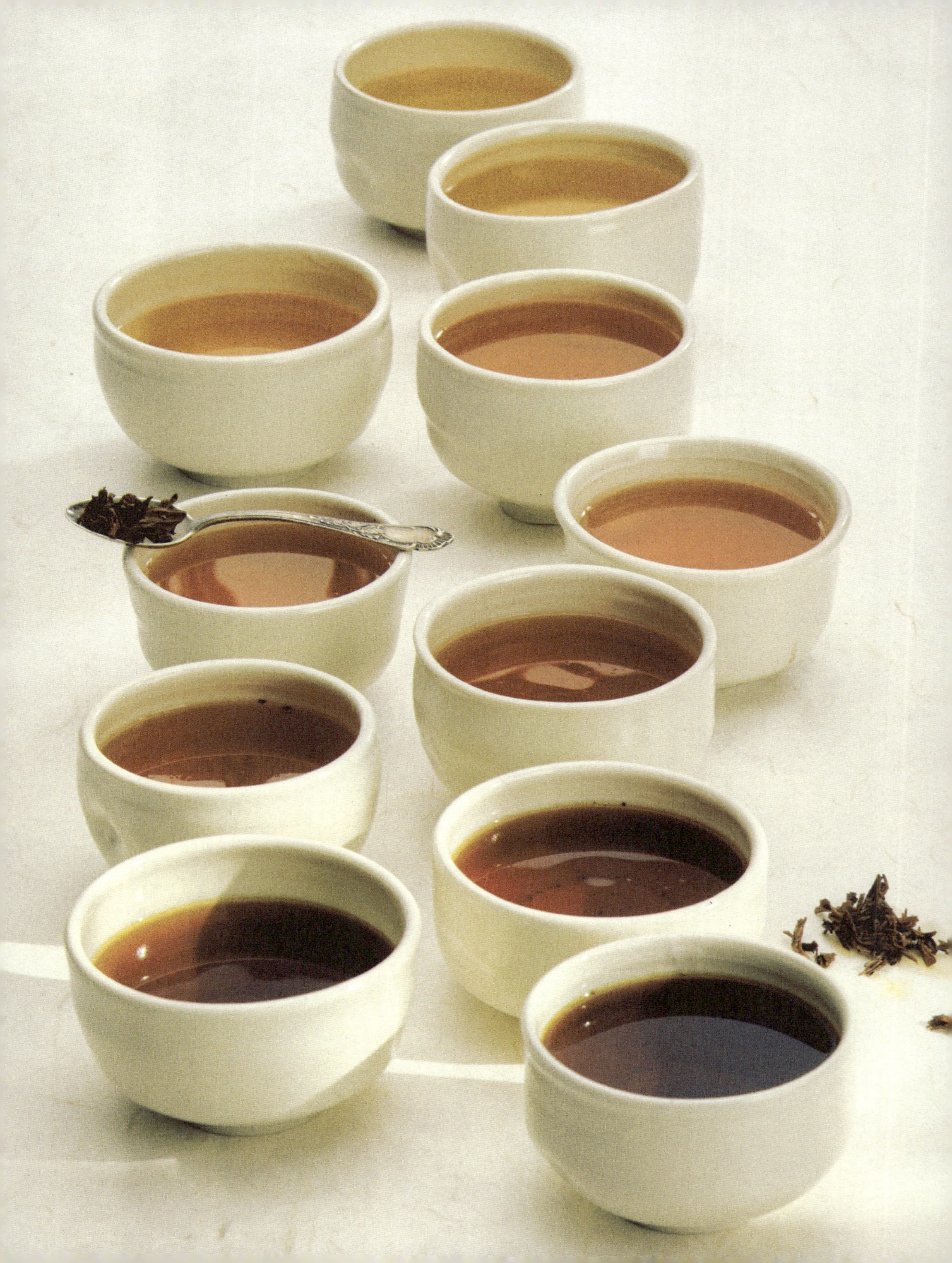

Black Tea Concentrate

ZAVARKA

Serves 4

Zavarka is basically a very strong black tea that you serve by pouring a small amount of it in a cup and topping it off with hot water. The small amount of concentrate becomes enough tea to flavor the rest of the water in the cup. This option, used often in Eastern European households, is really nice if you're having five to ten people over but don't have a large teapot. This way you can pour everybody a bit of tea from the teapot and then top their cups off with hot water. It's also a nice way to enjoy tea throughout the day without having to continuously empty out a teapot full of tea leaves. You can keep this concentrate for up to 24 hours.

Small teapot
Fine-mesh tea strainer

✣ ✣ ✣

2 tablespoons (4 to 6 g) loose black tea leaves

1 cup (240 ml) boiling water, preferably filtered, for the concentrate

Put the tea leaves in the teapot and pour the boiling water over the top. Let steep up to 12 hours; this is your concentrate. To serve, strain ¼ cup (60 ml) of the concentrated tea into a teacup. Then top off the cup using ¾ cup (177 ml) hot water.

NOTE: If you want to make more cups of tea, you can extrapolate the ratios from this recipe. For example, if you wanted to make 8 cups (1.9 l) of tea, you would use 4 tablespoons (8 to 12 g) tea leaves with 2 cups (480 ml) hot water poured over them and steeped for up to 12 hours.

What to Put in Black Tea

All teas can be enjoyed as they are, with nothing in them. But certain moments can call for the addition of sweeteners, citrus, or dairy. When it comes to dairy or lemon, use one or the other. The acidic flavor of lemon doesn't mix well with milk or cream.

MILK

Black tea, in particular, is high in tannins, a property that makes it pair well with milk. I love the comforting feeling that milk with black tea provides. I am partial to milky tea at night. The caffeine doesn't affect me and milk, tea, and honey comfort me before bed. If you are sensitive to caffeine, it's best not to drink it after two p.m. Another place for milk is in tea lattes, most often seen with matcha, but there are also Earl Grey lattes (London Fogs) or chai lattes that include warming spices like ginger, cardamom, or turmeric.

LEMON

Lemon creates a subtle tart flavor. In addition to the flavor, which is most popular for black tea, lemon has two other uses: first, it can be used with herbal teas to soothe the throat during cold and flu season; second, lemon in combination with tea can make the digestion-supportive properties of certain herbal teas stronger. Lemon can make bitter herbs more palatable, so it can aid in digestion if drinking bitters like yarrow, burdock, or even earthier flavors like echinacea.

SWEETENERS

As far as sweeteners go, the three most prevalent are sugar, maple syrup, and honey. Store-bought sugar is processed from sugarcane or sometimes beets. An advantage with sugar is its neutral flavor, but I prefer the raw sugar of maple syrup or honey. Maple syrup transports you to where it is tapped—in a dense forest—something lovely to think about while drinking tea. Raw honey tastes different depending on what plant the bees were pollinating, and I love tasting the variety. Honey also has antimicrobial and immune-supporting properties.

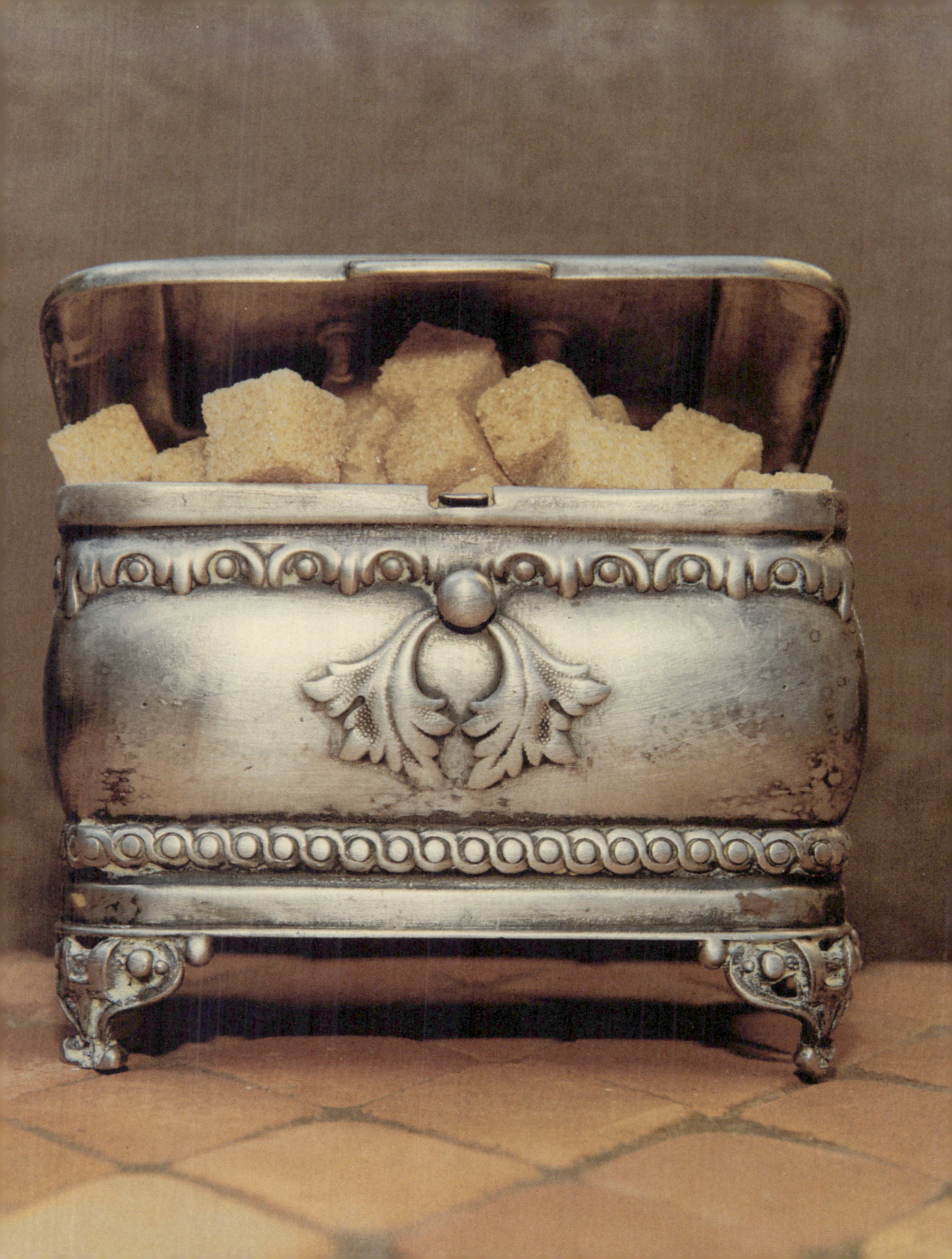

Green Tea

Serves 1

When making green tea, time and temperature are essential. Masha green teas are all grown in Japan, where tea leaves are steamed rather than roasted (I prefer the grassy, fresh taste of steamed green tea). Because of the delicate nature of steamed tea, our Japanese teas should be brewed for no more than one minute. Over brewing leads to acrid bitterness. For roasted green teas, like hōjicha, use the recipe for black tea (page 84).

Teapot

Electric kettle with temperature setting (optional)

Small fine-mesh tea strainer

Teacup

✢ ✢ ✢

About 1 teaspoon (3 g) loose sencha, kukicha, gyokuro, or genmaicha green tea leaves

1 cup (240 ml) water, preferably filtered

Place the tea in a teapot. Heat water to 160 to 175°F (71 to 80°C). If you don't have a thermometer, bring to just under a boil, or boil water and then let it cool for a few minutes. Pour the water over the tea in the teapot and steep for 1 minute (see Note). Strain into a teacup.

NOTE: Genmaicha, which is a sencha with toasted rice, can be brewed for 2 minutes total.

Herbal Tea

Serves 1

Herbal teas, also called tisanes, can be so forgiving. You can brew them for 3 to 5 minutes like black tea or you can infuse them for hours to get more of the effects of the herbs. For the most part, they don't get tannic when over brewed, though some can get bitter. If you're drinking Masha Calm Tea, a blend of lemon balm, chamomile, and calendula, at night you can definitely just make it in a few minutes, but if you want to get some of the calming properties of the herbs beyond just the tea ritual itself, I would let it sit longer—more like 10 or 15 minutes. For a lot of people, making infusions is a really effective and easy way to incorporate tea into daily life.

When drinking herbal tea for the flavor alone, use this recipe for a simple cup of herbal tea. To make an herbal blend of leaves or flowers for medicinal purposes, use the herbal infusions recipe; to make a medicinal blend of roots or seeds, use the herbal decoctions recipe (these recipes follow). Please note that the density of different herbs can vary. If you don't have a kitchen scale, know that you will use a smaller amount of an herb that is finely milled and more of an herb that is coarsely milled.

Teapot

Electric kettle with temperature setting (optional)

Fine-mesh tea strainer

Teacup

About 1 teaspoon finely milled herb or
4 teaspoons of a full-leaf, lighter herb (3 g)

1 cup (240 ml) water, preferably filtered

Place the tea in a teapot. Heat water to 190 to 212°F (boiling) [88 to 100°C]. Pour the boiling water over the herbs in the teapot and steep for 5 to 10 minutes. Strain into a teacup.

Herbal Infusions

Serves 1

1 heaping tablespoon (about 14 g) dried herbal tea (flowers and leaves) *or* 3 tablespoons (about 5 g) chopped fresh herbs (flowers and leaves)

1 cup (240 ml) water, preferably filtered

Put the herbs in a teapot. Heat water to 190 to 212°F (boiling) [88 to 100°C]. Pour the boiling water over the herbs in the teapot. Cover the pot and let the tea sit for 10 to 15 minutes. Strain into a teacup.

Herbal Decoctions

Serves 1

1 tablespoon (14 g) dried herbal tea (roots, barks, rhizomes, and seeds) *or* 3 tablespoons (5 g) fresh herbs (roots, barks, rhizomes, and seeds)

1 cup (240 ml) water, preferably filtered

Combine the dried or fresh herbs and the water in a small saucepan and bring to a boil. Cover the saucepan and simmer for 20 minutes. Remove the saucepan from the heat and let steep for an additional 10 minutes. Strain into a teacup and serve.

Brewing Time and Temperature

black	3 to 5 minutes	190 to 212°F (88 to 100°C)
green	1 to 2 minutes*	160 to 175°F (71 to 80°C)
herbal (leaves, flowers, seeds, and roots)	5 to 15 minutes	190 to 212°F (88 to 100°C)
oolong	3 to 5 minutes	185 to 200°F (85 to 93°C)
white	2 to 3 minutes	160 to 175°F (71 to 80°C)

* When blending green tea, or when brewing blends like genmaicha, which is green tea with toasted rice, it's okay to brew it for a few extra minutes.

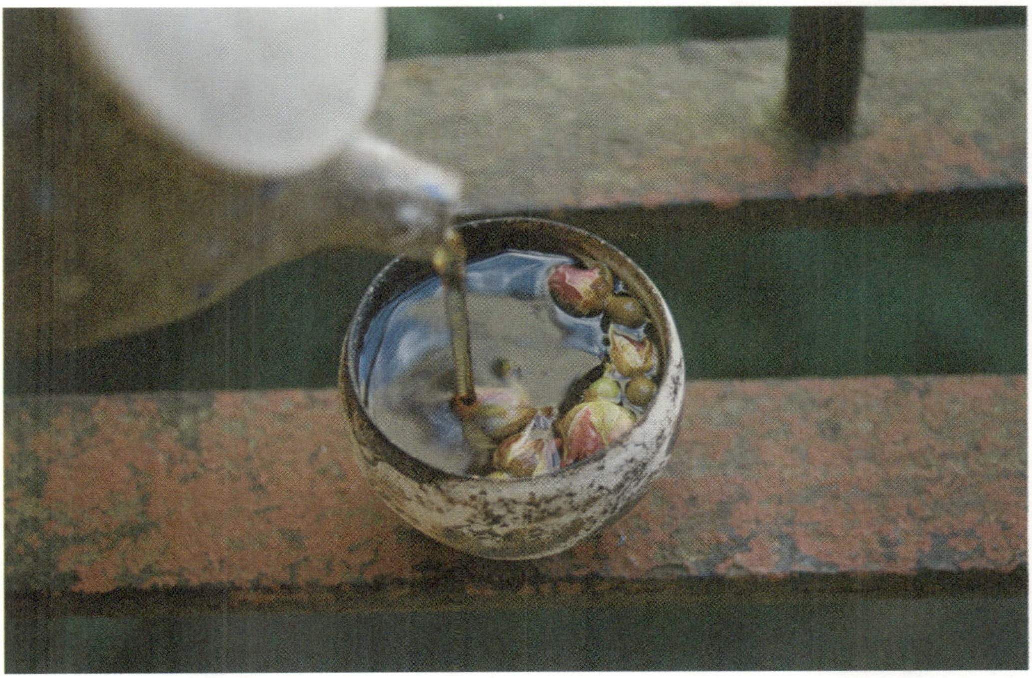

Cold Brew

Makes 6 cups

This is the easiest iced tea recipe to make—and the best part is that you make it overnight so it's ready in the morning! Brewing tea with cold water brings out different properties than hot water. Green teas, for example, are typically less tannic and bitter when cold-brewed. Something like the Masha Love Tea looks really pretty floating around in a glass jar because of the organic roses, organic anise hyssop, and eastern red cedar. Any tea that can be prepared hot can also be cold-brewed.

64-ounce (1.9 l) mason jar

Fine-mesh tea strainer

3 tablespoons (about 8 g) tea leaves
(and/or herbal roots, seeds, or flowers)

Room temperature or cold water, preferably filtered

Ice (optional)

Put the herbs in the mason jar, fill with the water, and screw on the lid. Let steep for at least 6 hours and up to overnight in the fridge. If making during the day, you can shake the jar every few hours to move the herbs around (and to enjoy the snow globe effect). You can serve as is or over ice. Place a strainer over a large cup, fill with ice (if using), and strain the tea into it.

NOTE: You can make Tea over Ice by bringing 1 cup (240 ml) water to 190 to 212°F (boiling) [88 to 100°C] for black and herbal tea, or 160 to 175°F (71 to 80°C) for green tea. Place 2 heaping teaspoons (6 g) loose tea leaves in a teapot and pour in the hot water. Let sit for about 5 minutes for black or herbal tea or 1 to 2 minutes for green tea. Fill a heat-resistant, shatterproof cup with about 1 cup (220 g) ice. Strain directly over the ice.

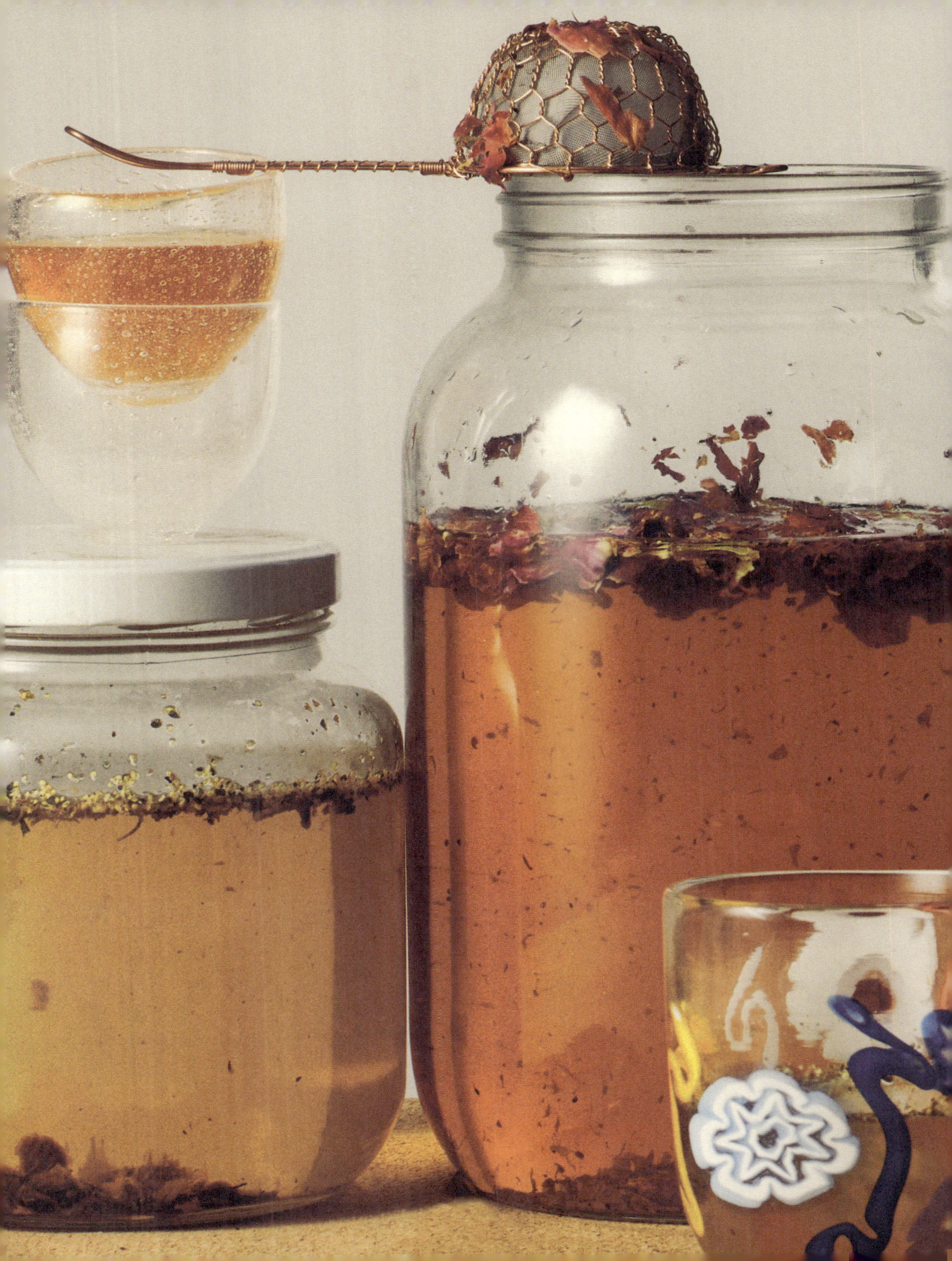

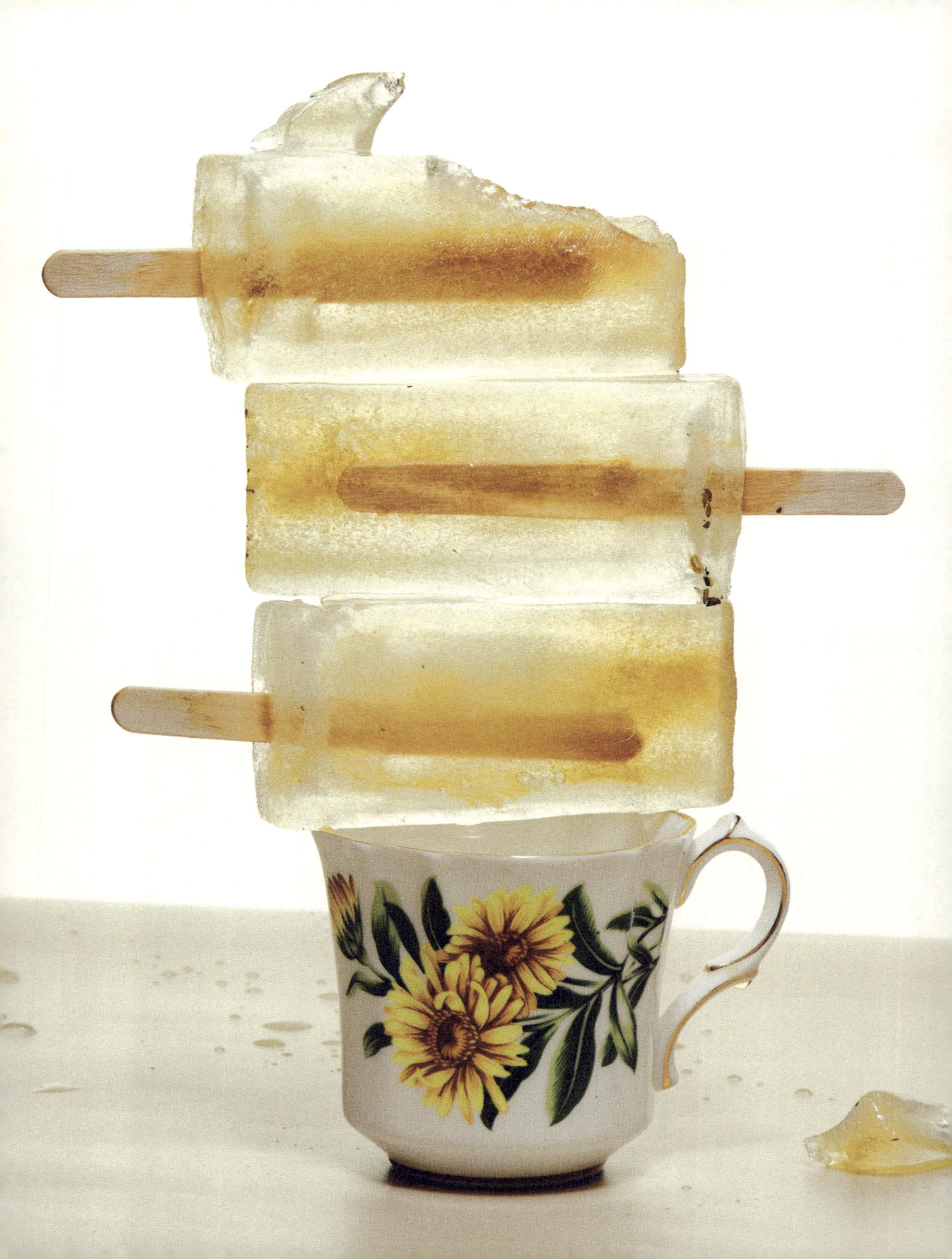

Tea Ice Pops

Makes 6

In the summer, I always have ice pops in the freezer, made from fresh fruit, tea, or both. Licorice tea makes a great base for ice pops because it is so naturally sweet and cooling. I love to make iced tea ice pops with a Masha Tea blend called Après, which contains mint, fennel, and licorice. If you want to add some texture, place half a teaspoon of fennel seeds into each ice pop, or blend in whatever fruit you have on hand—I like cantaloupe, watermelon, and berries.

32-ounce (950 ml) glass jar

Teapot

Fine-mesh tea strainer

Funnel

6 metal ice pop molds

6 ice pop sticks

✢ ✢ ✢

1 tablespoon (2 to 3 g) herbal tea (you can use Après tea or any blend of your choosing)

2 cups (480 ml) water, preferably filtered, at room temperature

Place the herbs in the glass jar and pour the water over the herbs. To cold-brew the tea, put the jar in the fridge overnight. The next morning, or at least 6 hours later, strain the tea into a measuring cup or teapot. Pour the tea into the molds. Freeze for at least 6 hours or overnight. Run the molds under warm water if you're having trouble removing the ice pops.

Matcha

The process of making matcha is one of inherent thoughtfulness because it's prepared in a stepwise fashion. You can't check your phone while whisking, and it's mesmerizing to watch bright green tea mix slowly into creamy milk. I recommend refrigerating high-quality matcha to preserve freshness and color. If you're not sure about the quality of the matcha that you're using, take a bit and spread it out on white paper. What is the color like? The consistency? Ideally, the matcha that you're buying is bright green and smooth. Is it certified organic? Sometimes, farmers who are practicing organic agriculture may not have the finances or desire to obtain certification. As with any tea or agricultural product, you can always chat with the supplier about sourcing practices.

Matcha has been at the heart of Japanese tea ceremony for centuries; people trained for years, and still do, to prepare it properly. But it has also transformed into the go-to café order of today. Some consider it a more mindful alternative as a home routine to preparing coffee. Matcha, in Japanese tea ceremony, is prepared with just water and matcha powder. No milk. It is served with *wagashi* (artful tea candies that are an art of their own to prepare). The creation of matcha lattes, incorporating milk into the traditionally somewhat bitter drink to sweeten it and make it more appealing to the masses, is contemporary. Luckily, it is delicious and easy to make at home.

Many milk alternatives exist for those who prefer not to drink cow's milk (though I personally think that the best lattes are made with whole milk). Milk from oat, pistachio, almond, soy, walnut, cashew—the list goes on—can all be used in hot or iced matcha lattes, and it is truly a matter of personal preference. I find that a lot of the store-bought milk alternatives have gums and other preservatives in them that can lead to digestive upset. For that reason, the best nut milks and milk alternatives are made at home, or bought fresh at a local food coop.

Hot Matcha Latte

Serves 1

Electric kettle with temperature setting (optional)

Instant-read thermometer

Heat-resistant cup

Electric milk steamer (optional)

Tea scoop (or a teaspoon if you don't have one)

Small fine-mesh strainer (for sifting)

Chawan (a tea bowl, or any small bowl will do if you don't have one dedicated to matcha)

Matcha whisk

✢ ✢ ✢

2 tablespoons water, preferably filtered

1 cup (240 ml) milk

1 teaspoon (3 g) matcha powder

Heat the water to 160 to 175°F (71 to 80°C) and transfer it to a heat-resistant cup to cool down. Warm up the milk to about 285 to 320°F (140 to 160°C). If doing this on the stove, cook it at very low heat so it doesn't come to a boil. Alternatively, consider investing in a milk steamer. Sift the matcha into a tea bowl. Pour some hot water over the matcha powder, just enough to cover it. Whisk the matcha and hot water. You'll know you're done whisking when bubbles form at the surface. This should happen in about 20 to 30 seconds. Pour the warm milk into a heat-resistant cup. Pour the matcha over the warm milk and enjoy.

Iced Matcha

Serves 1

I went through a phase of buying bodega ice for daily iced matcha lattes at home. Eventually, I bought an ice-cube tray. The caffeine content of matcha, while high, tends to create a more balanced energy than the sometimes-frenetic feel generated by an afternoon coffee.

12-ounce (350 ml) heat-resistant cup

Tea scoop (or a teaspoon if you don't have one)

Small fine-mesh strainer (for sifting)

Chawan (tea bowl, or any small bowl will do if you don't have one)

Matcha whisk

✣ ✣ ✣

2 tablespoons water, preferably filtered

Ice (enough to fill your cup)

1 cup (240 ml) milk

1 teaspoon (3 g) matcha powder

Heat the water to 160 to 175°F (71 to 80°C). Fill a heat-resistant cup with ice then fill three-fourths of the cup with milk. Sift matcha into a bowl. Pour in enough hot water to cover the matcha. Whisk the matcha and water for 30 seconds. Pour the matcha mixture over the ice and milk.

NOTE: It's true that there is a meticulous way to make matcha, and that Japanese tea masters dedicate decades of their lives to perfecting this art. But remember, there is no right or wrong way when it comes to making tea at home. Enjoy the beauty and the imperfections. The key to becoming somebody who drinks tea regularly is to drink tea regularly. The how finds a way of working itself out.

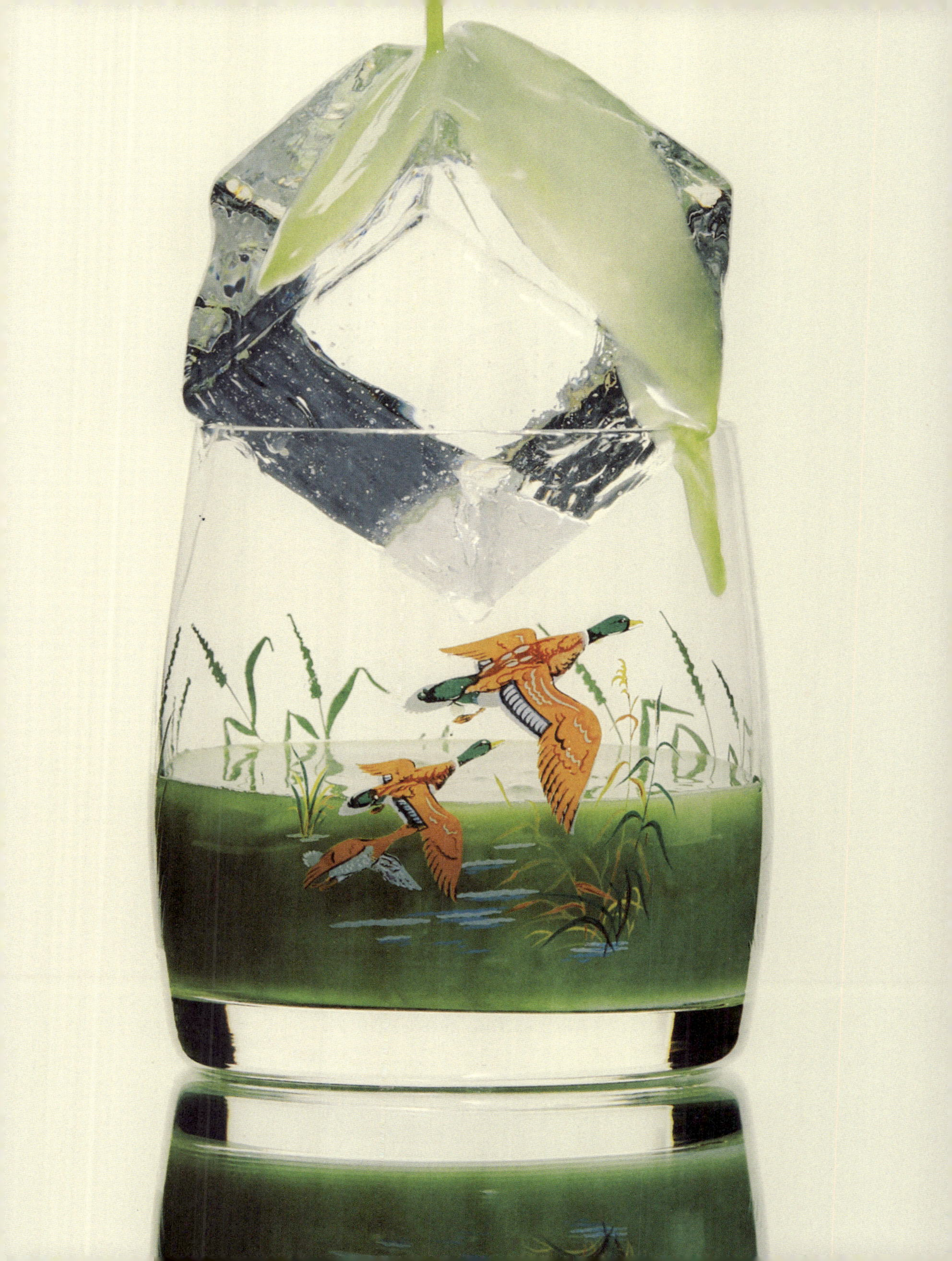

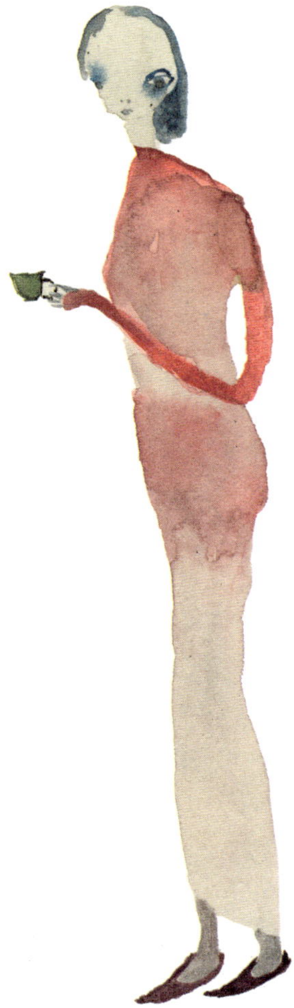

"Every day is all there is."
—Joan Didion,
New York Times interview (1977)

– 7 –

Establishing a Tea Ritual

We're really interested, as a culture, in the routines and habits of famous people, athletes, and even writers (Joan Didion notoriously had a Coke and a cigarette every morning). We're curious about the day-to-day of people we deem interesting or successful. I think we want to know these things because we wonder if we changed our own habits and routines would we too change? Would we become more interesting and successful ourselves?

But copying somebody else's routine will not create a better version of you. It's more important to focus instead on a personalized combination of habits and established routines.

The concept of ritual—something that is done habitually with intention—and its application to tea can be extrapolated from the examples provided in this chapter. Tea rituals can, and have, been a part of myriad lifestyles and cultures. For creative, busy people, developing a ritual around tea is a simple way to add rest, beauty, and purpose into the everyday.

A tea ritual can be a way for families to spend time together, all using the same cups and herbs, having a shared experience. A tea ritual can also be a way to connect with yourself and your creativity. The best way to begin a new ritual or routine is to just start doing it, one day at a time.

Why a Tea Ritual

Drinking tea can put you in touch with yourself. If you are present, calm, nonreactive, this is when the best decisions happen, the most fated accidental encounters. Drinking tea every day puts you in the mindset of that possibility. It doesn't mean that every day is necessarily mindful or peaceful or magical, but that your body has a baseline and the muscle memory to get there. Tea is a gentle way to regulate how we feel; when you drink tea every day with intention, it becomes a ritual that can profoundly impact daily life.

What a Tea Ritual Looks Like

A ritual can be about a time of day: a morning ritual could include a nourishing breakfast with tea, or it can be about the thing itself, a tea ritual. There are ways to mark a ritual, using scent, for example, like lighting a candle or burning incense. In the case of tea, scent is inherent in the ritual itself. A ritual has a beginning and end. In the case of a tea ritual, it may begin with pouring water into a kettle and it may end with washing a cup. A tea ritual might mean going to the same café every afternoon to order a matcha, or it could mean taking thirty minutes in the evening to make an herbal tea and to journal. A ritual should express elements of beauty, thoughtfulness, and care. By creating time to appreciate beauty and to consider what we may need to feel cared for in the future, we show ourselves self-respect and value. A tea ritual is an accessible way to bring these simple luxuries into daily life. There are various approaches to determining which tea to incorporate into your ritual. To begin, select one to three teas to rotate so that you don't get overwhelmed. Eventually, you might have something like a "house" tea, which for me is holy basil. It's a tea that I always have at my home that I know most others don't have. So when I'm including other people in my rituals, it's a tea that I love to share with them.

To initiate a new ritual, begin with what you have available. Rather than focusing on acquiring the perfect tools, consider how to be creative with the tools and teas that you already have, even if it's a pot of boiling water on the stove and a tea bag from the grocery store. Meanwhile, you can fill in the gaps, and get the strainer and the beautiful teacup, the kettle, and the teapot, but the actual ritual itself does not hinge on those material aspects.

Establishing a ritual of any kind is predicated on just starting and continuing it—daily, seasonally, or annually, depending on the nature of the ritual. Once you start, make a commitment to yourself.

One effective way to start would be to pair drinking tea with an activity that you do every day and enjoy: it might be related to skincare, exercise, or any similar daily activity that makes you feel good. Tea before or after would be a simple way to establish a tea ritual based around something you're doing that already feels good. Perhaps you have a weekly ritual of going to the farmers market or grocery store: choosing something that could accompany your tea, or be blended into it, can keep the tea ritual fresh and interesting.

Perhaps more simply, though, tea is so lovely when shared with others. It doesn't need to be more complicated than that. You can have your morning tea ritual and create added excitement and joy by working tea into your life in other ways at other times, like making a pot to share with a parent, sibling, or new friend. Doing so offers a moment of connection, and those moments with others can strengthen the rituals that we do alone.

Morning Tea for One

Caffeine, whether in the form of black tea, matcha, or coffee, is the way many people around the world start their mornings. A boost of energy, an awakening, the way that we enter our mornings sets the tone for the rest of the day. The first meal and drink of the day should be something that you know will make you feel healthy, full, and energized. Later in the day, we're more susceptible to cravings, to impulse, to whims, and because of that, the morning is an easy time to establish a routine that feels healthy. I love to have tea with fruit and yogurt or cottage cheese for breakfast and have some version of this almost every day. Morning coffee drinkers could try a month of having black tea or matcha in the morning instead of coffee—many people find that tea is gentler than coffee and lowers anxiety throughout the day.

Tea with a Friend

Tea and long conversations with a friend go hand in hand. Consider choosing a tea that you can easily rebrew. Green teas are great for this. After you brew it and pour it into cups, you can have a pot of hot water ready to pour over the leaves for a second brew, and continue for multiple brews. For the most success with rebrewing, use tiny cups and a small teapot. Another approach is the opposite—to use enormous mugs, so that you can keep the warm, comforting cup of tea in hand over a long period of conversation. In that case, you can start with one tea and, after a while, you can take a break to intentionally make another kind. As for the types of tea to drink, having a friend over is the best time to try out a new or special blend, or to share something they may not have tried before.

Tea in the Afternoon

Afternoon tea exists for a reason. We all often need a pick-me-up at around three p.m., whether in the form of caffeine, a break from hours of working, or simply to acknowledge the turn of the day toward evening. If you are someone who is trying to cut down on coffee, the afternoon is a great time to switch to matcha or green tea to still get a caffeine boost without also getting jittery. If you don't drink caffeine after the morning, include adaptogenic teas like holy basil or licorice to keep your mood balanced and steady.

Tea in the Evening

In a world that is hyper-stimulating, at times overwhelming and stressful, sleep often eludes us. Creating a ritual before bed can signal to our systems that it's time to wind down. Part of an evening ritual can be a shower, brushing teeth, a skincare routine, and a cup of tea. An herbal tea acts on our physiology to calm us, but there's also an intentional process required, albeit a quick one. Choosing a teapot and cup, putting the water on to boil, handling the tea. It's a conversation with someone you live with about what kind of tea they want, a grounding into the present moment, which in this case is a quiet closing to the day. Moments in time can be used to establish a ritual.

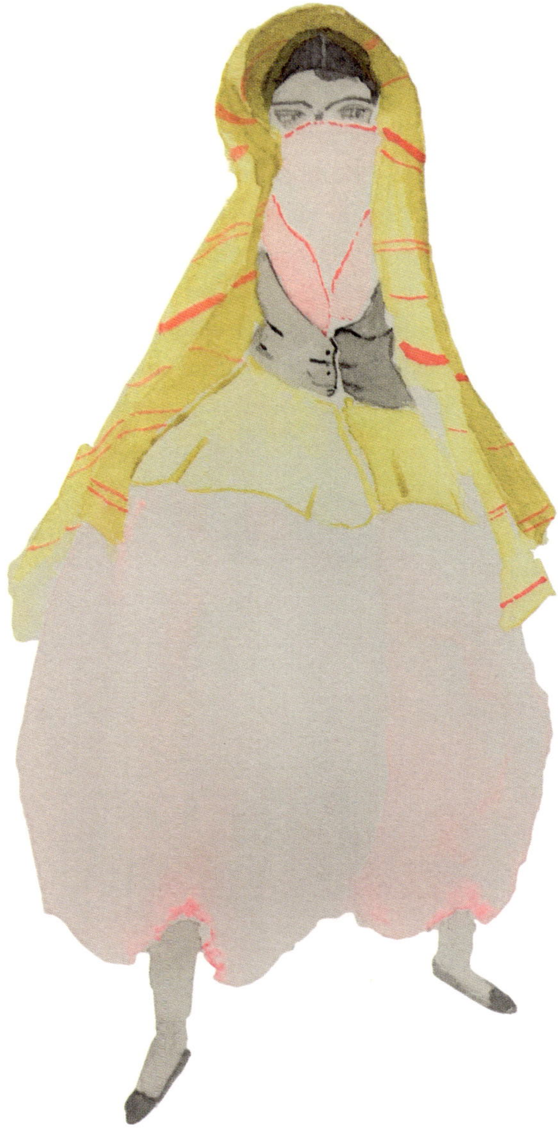

Tea with a Partner

"Picture me upon your knee
Just tea for tea and two for tea."
—Irving Caesar and Vincent Youmans,
"Tea for Two" (1924)

What are rituals when it comes to romance? We don't think of romance as ritualistic, yet are there not rituals in the preparation for first dates, in putting on makeup or shaving, in holding open a door for a date? As the dance of romance develops into a relationship, we establish rituals with a partner: one person may prepare tea, another breakfast. Intentionally incorporating tea into romance rituals can lead to intimacy. Tea tends to be innocent, grounding, calming, and beautiful, and can help you actually get to know somebody. It can also be an innocuous and unassuming way to

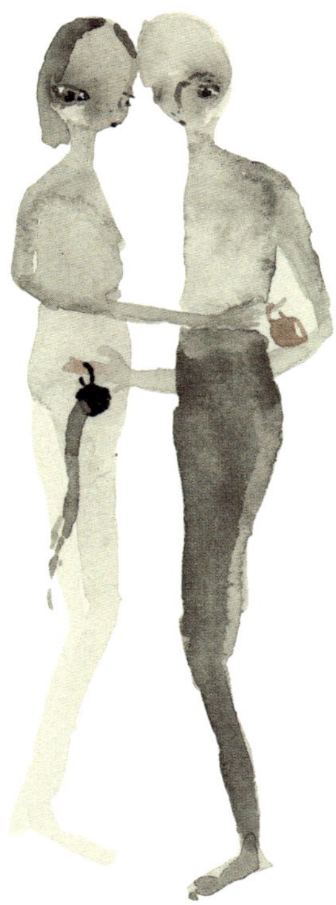

invite someone into your space to talk after a date without the implications of alcohol. Tea is subtler. A glass of wine or a drink suggests a loosening or a change in your state of mind. Tea is kind of the opposite: it might connotate a sharpening of focus or a way to wind down toward the end of an evening, but still staying true to yourself. Though of course tea also can be a great base for cocktails.

Making a cup of tea for somebody signifies generosity and care without being over-the-top, and it's charming. The element of lighting a candle with an evening tea or sharing a small snack can also be so cute, and a way to show an element of your personal style. When getting to know somebody romantically, you want there to be ease, honesty, and calm—all attributes brought out by a simple cup of tea.

Romance can be an impetus for establishing a ritual. On this note, all weddings should have a tea component. Iced tea is such a simple nonalcoholic option to have at the bar. It could otherwise be tea and coffee with dessert or a breakfast moment the morning after. To make this thoughtful, choose tea and coffee brands that speak to the space or style of the wedding location and couple. Ideally, the brands are either local to the wedding venue or local to a special place in the couple's history. Packaged tea also makes for a lovely wedding favor.

Like the Leonard Cohen song implies, being invited over for tea can be a transformative experience.

Tea for Celebrations

Whether it's the changing of the seasons, religious or cultural holidays, annual celebrations can be a way to create meaningful rituals. Knowing that your family hosts a particular holiday every year, you can choose one dish to keep consistent and the rest can be up for change. This is also a great excuse to have an extra set of teacups to serve many guests, to incorporate a tea course with a signature dessert, and to choose seasonal teas. For winter holidays, serve tea with individual cinnamon sticks or star anise. Incorporate fresh herbs into floral arrangements as well as into tea blends to create visual and taste relationships with seasonal teas. It's fun to be the person who brings and makes tea for the group.

Tea and Creativity

Tea can be part of a creative ritual. If you are a writer or an artist, it can be helpful to establish a sensory space to work within. Maybe making a cup of tea marks that you are about to start working.

I have kept a journal since the third grade. I remember choosing a puffy little diary with a tiny lock and key from a small book fair at my elementary school. For the majority of my life, I have carried a journal with me everywhere I go. I don't write in it every day, and I don't have a set time to write. Some people establish journaling rituals by doing it that way—writing every morning at the same table, for example. In college, I had a little spot by a big window in my dorm that I called the tea corner. It looked out to the forest, and I would put a bunch of pillows and blankets on the floor there. I loved getting cozy in that corner, looking out the floor-to-ceiling window, with my giant mug of tea in hand. I can remember the mug now: it was oversize ceramic with a pink and brown pattern. I spent so many hours at that window drinking tea and writing in my journal. I wrote about boys, and classes, but mostly I wrote about my relationship with myself, and my growing self-awareness as a young woman. I made up my mind to study abroad in India in that corner, and wrote about the excitement of the anticipation, all with my cup of tea in hand.

Years later in Brooklyn, I remember one summer when each day the first thing I did was go out to the park near my apartment, by the river, and sit on a blanket while leaning against a brick wall and journal. It was one of the pandemic summers and I was living alone. Rituals like journaling made me feel grateful that I was in New York during the pandemic. As a single person at the time, my neighborhood felt like a community and I loved being able to see people going about their days. It made me feel grounded.

Through these times and experiences, I have continued to carry my journal with me all over the city, and the world. Having a journal with me at all times is a habit that I established as a teenager and have kept. The ritual for me is having the journal with me. I take it out when I have a moment alone at a café, while waiting at the airport, sitting in a park, or if I just need to calm myself.

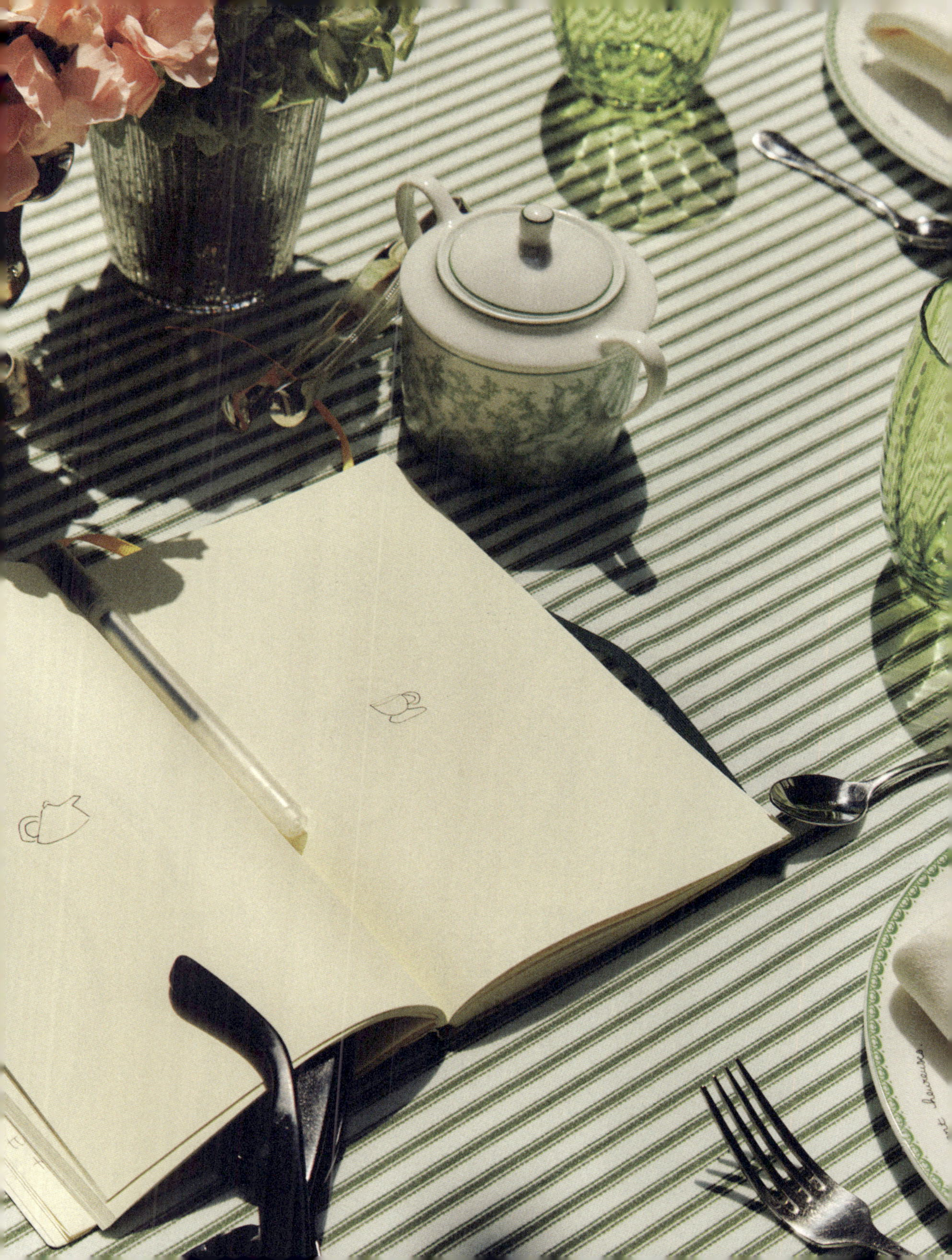

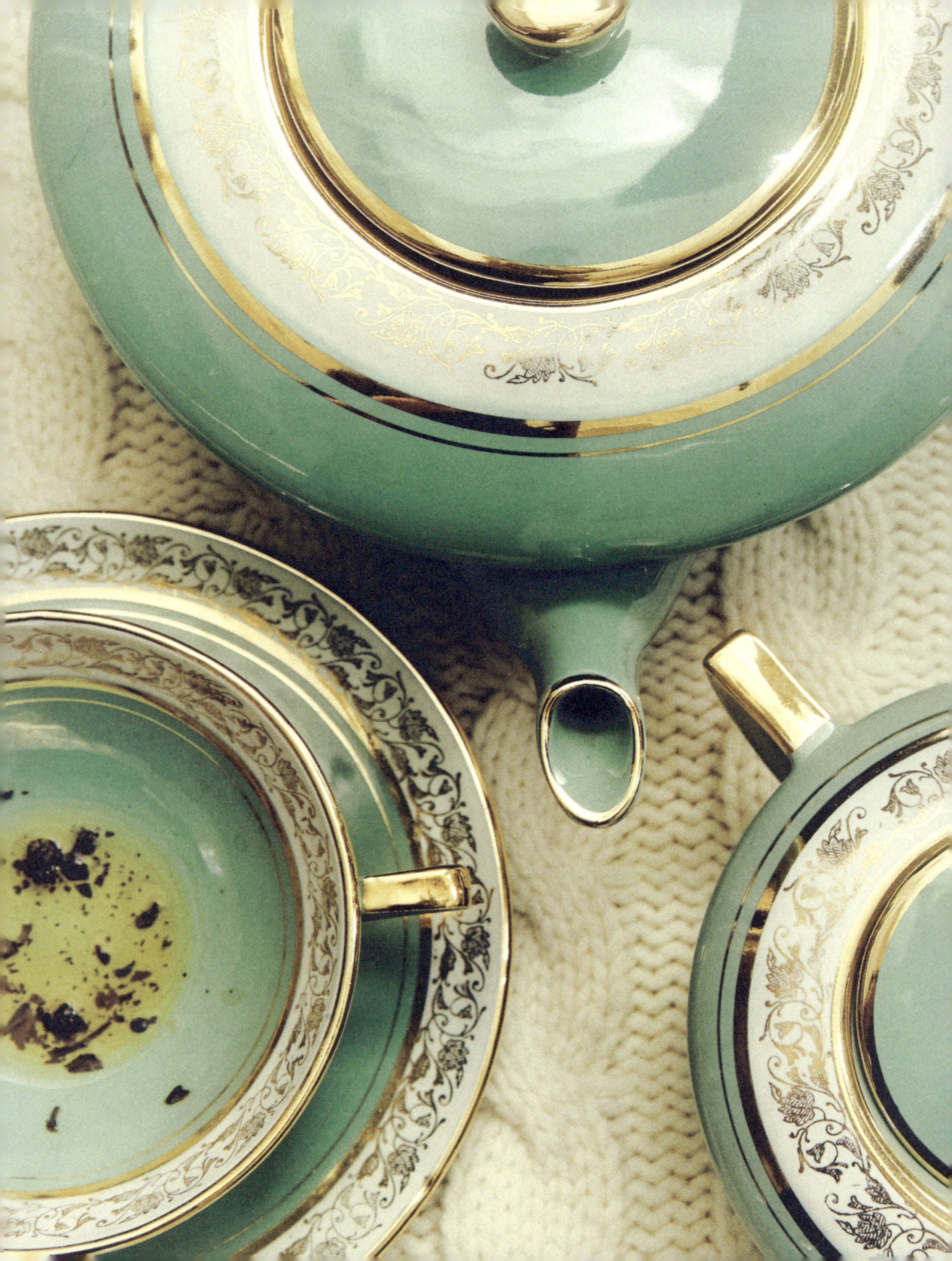

Mystical Rituals: Reading Tea Leaves

> "A keen interest in any form of divination is the inevitable result of uncertain times, all in the hope that some glimmer of light might brighten the darkness and obscurity of the future."
>
> —The Highland Seer,
> *Reading Tea Leaves*, 1920

Tasseomancy, from the French word *tasse* for cup and from the Greek *manteia*, meaning prophecy, refers to the practice of reading tea leaves.

The tasseomancy tome is a Scottish text called *Reading Tea Leaves*, released in 1920 by "The Highland Seer," who writes that tea-leaf reading is horary, meaning it foretells events in the coming hours, or a full day at most, "even if the student doesn't deeply believe in the accuracy of what he sees in the cup, reading of the tea leaves is a fun diversion for the breakfast table."

Tea-leaf reading is best performed with full-leaf green tea, in a cup that is wide on top and not too narrow on the bottom, so that symbols can be seen clearly. The inside should be white, without any prints.

First prepare a cup of tea with unstrained tea leaves and drink most of it, leaving just a tablespoon or so on the bottom. Using the left hand, swirl the cup three times clockwise, then place it upside down over the saucer so the water drains out. Once the water has drained, the cup can be picked up and the tea leaves are ready to read.

Evaluating the tea leaves is "a bit like seeing pictures in the clouds," but a list has been compiled over the years, with symbols of good fortune including stars, triangles, trees, bridges, and flowers, and symbols of bad fortune including clouds, umbrellas, snakes, swords, owls, and monkeys. Pigeons can indicate important news if they're flying, and if at rest, they can mean "domestic bliss and wealth acquired in trade."

It's human nature to look for the divine in the everyday, and the way that tea can make us feel—comfortable, at peace, relaxed—makes it clear why mystics turned, and continue to turn, toward a simple cup of tea for information about what the present and future hold.

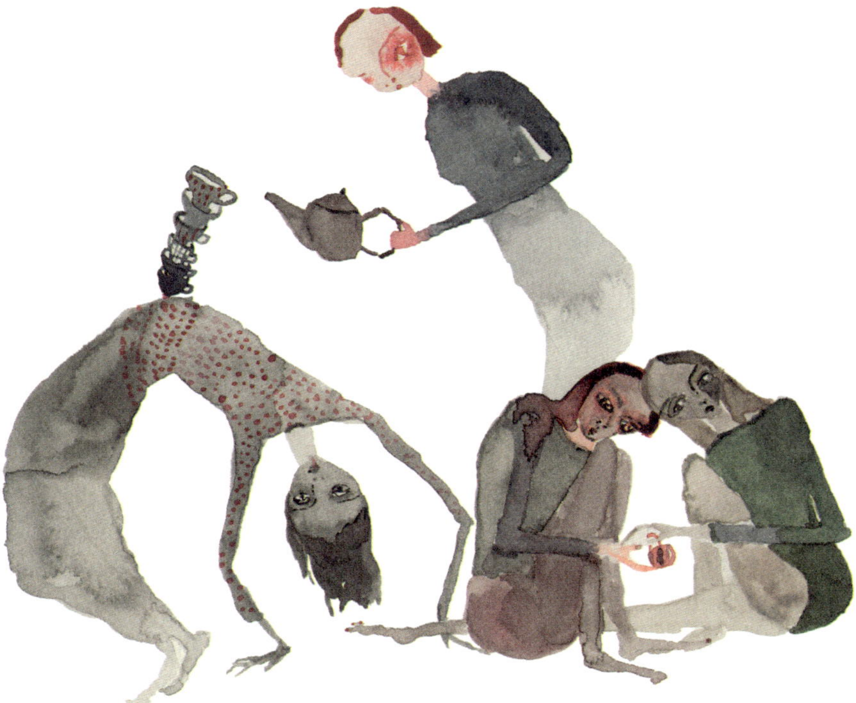

"After an evening spent with the Lopezes, my father would come home exalting to the high heavens their apartment, their furniture, the tea served in beautiful porcelain cups from a trolley. He would say Frances was 'in the know,' meaning she knew where to find nice furniture and beautiful cups, she knew how to decorate a home and how to serve tea."

—Natalia Ginzburg, *Family Lexicon*

(2017)

– 8 –

Tea and Hosting

Hosting is all about creating an atmosphere. A comfortable atmosphere might mean cozy, romantic, elegant, laid-back—even professional, depending on the occasion. The best way to be a great host is to feel confident, unrushed, and at ease with yourself, and to serve tea and food that you personally enjoy. I've hosted people for tea on the floor in apartments that don't have furniture yet with water I boiled on the stovetop, and I've hosted ticketed multicourse dinners alongside incredible chefs with each course paired with tea. If you have tea and a story to tell, you can host tea at home. Now that you have the confidence to serve tea, I'll walk you through some considerations, from cups to lighting, around how to do it well.

When serving tea with dessert after a dinner, make it easy for yourself to prepare tea for the number of guests. The simplest approach is to choose one to three teas to make. In my home, I always make black tea and I usually have one or two herbal options as well. I like to put teapots on the table—one with black tea and one with herbal—for visual effect and for guests to serve themselves. If the teapot does not have a built-in strainer, don't forget to put a little plate with a strainer on the table. Think about the number of cups of tea your teapots hold and determine how many teapots you'll need based on that. For seconds, you can always rebrew the tea leaves by pouring hot water over them a second time. Another option for serving black tea to a large party is to make a concentrate (see concentrate recipe, page 87). Depending on the number of people, I put out one or two saucers of milk, a dish or two with cut lemons, and a pot or two of honey on each end of the table alongside dessert.

Some other dining customs that I've carried over from my Eastern European heritage are superstitions. You should never hug, kiss, or shake hands through a doorway, so I always step out or wait for guests to come fully in before embracing. People who sit at the corner of a table will never get married, so children or single guests should not be seated at corners (it's uncomfortable anyway, and not a reasonable place to seat somebody, but sometimes you need to make space!). And applicable to those traveling long distances, before leaving for a long trip, everybody present (whether going on the trip or not) sits down and sits silently for several minutes to ensure a safe return home.

Choosing Tea for Hosting

You should have one or two teas that you love that are easy, go-to teas for you, so whenever you have someone over, you are able to offer one tea and one herbal option. Decide if you are more of a green or black tea household. Personally, I live in a black tea household; it's a classic for me. For the herbal option, mint and chamomile are easy. Beyond your two basic teas, you can start to build out a tea drawer or tea cabinet. I love to pick up tea when I travel, especially to tea-growing countries. I think about buying tea for home the same way that I think about sourcing tea for Masha Tea—choosing elevated classics, thoughtful blends, and delicious herbs. Create a tea menu based on the number of guests you will have. For something like a cheese board, you might have two to three cheeses if you just have a couple of guests over and more like five to six if it's many people. For food that guests serve themselves, it's great to have many options and an abundance in quantity. The number of teas that you serve is the opposite. With tea, you want to serve it hot and ideally to everyone almost at once. When you're dealing with loose tea, making even just one kind of tea for a big group can be time-consuming and cumbersome, so you want to make it as easy for yourself as possible; for a smaller group, you can have several options available. The fewer kinds of tea you make for a big group, the easier it will be. Choose tea that you like and can speak to and start small. For a very large party, high-quality tea bags can be super helpful—all you need to do is have water ready. Guests can pour their own water over the tea bags if you put the kettle on the table.

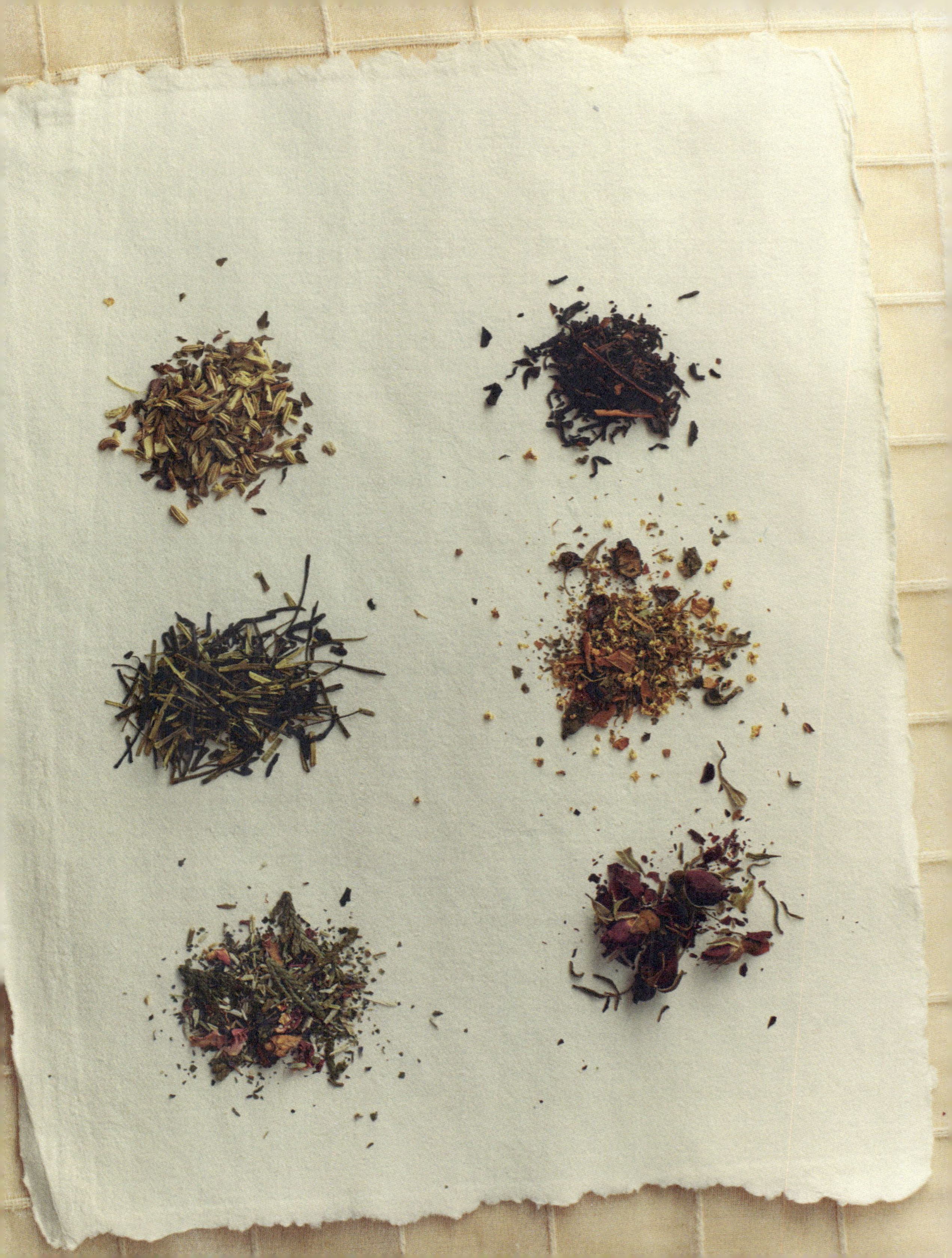

Choosing Teapots and Teacups

At home, I have several teapots that hold anywhere from one to ten cups of tea, and I choose the appropriate size teapot depending on how many guests I have over. For larger gatherings, if you're not using tea bags, it is convenient to have two large teapots so that you can always brew two different types of tea at a time for the table. A smaller teapot can be really intimate when making tea for just a couple of people, especially if you have tiny teacups to match. You can spend an entire evening brewing and rebrewing a pot of tea and sharing tea from the tiny cups with a friend. For an evening gathering, when tea is served after dinner, it's okay to make enough for guests to have at least one cup with dessert, but it's always good hosting to have more. After the first teapots are empty, make a second batch for the table.

Another consideration is straining the tea leaves. Some teapots have built-in mesh strainers, other ceramic ones have holes built into the ceramics, and others have no built-in strainer at all. The former works for all kinds of tea, no matter how small the tea leaves are sifted and cut. The cut-outs in ceramic teapots are great for whole-leaf tea, but sometimes allow smaller herbs through. For those and for teapots without built-in strainers, you need a way to strain the leaves (see infusers, page 78).

When hosting, consider creating an element of choice in teacups. I have five cups from a set that I like to use—each one differs in color and pattern—and I love to let people pick their own and see which they decide on. If you don't have a mismatched tea set but are using handmade ceramics, or even diner mugs, you can create the same experience of choice for people. At one point, I had collected so many mugs that before a dinner and tea that I hosted for a large group of fifteen guests, I pruned one of my house plants and put a cutting of the plant with water in each of the mugs. I put them all in my claw-foot bathtub. When guests left for the night, they were invited to go and choose a plant and mug to take home with them and replant in their own apartments. As a guest, I love being asked to pick my own cup or mug. I think it's a fun and sweet moment. If a guest says they don't care, it's also interesting to consider what they might like, such as a particular pattern, an ironic mug, or a cup with a backstory, for example.

Hosting a Dinner Party

I found a mirror of my childhood meals in Brooklyn, and of my hosting style today, in Darra Goldstein's book, *A La Russe: A Cookbook of Russian Hospitality* (1983), about her time living in the Soviet Union and the food and customs of the people she met. She writes about how hosts always had samovars with hot water ready to serve, about many people seated around a dining table in the largest room of a small apartment, of neighbors dropping in, the host busying themselves making tea, the abundant desserts, and cognac, wine, and vodka lingering on the table even when the tea is gone.

This was the dining experience at my grandmother's Brooklyn apartment when I was growing up, and it is the experience that I create in my own apartment when hosting dinners, one that I am realizing extends to tsarist Russia. I like to fit as many people as possible around the table, with old friends and new sitting side by side. With parties of more than six, I make place cards and choose seating intentionally. I do this to encourage both friendship and interesting conversation. Guests always get the most comfortable seats, but even within that, I try to consider each individual and which dishes they might want to be sitting near, and which view of the room might be compelling for them.

Eastern European meals begin with a *zakuski* course, similar to charcuterie or hors d'oeuvres. Zakuski are cold appetizers, such as caviar, deviled eggs, crudités, pickles, and cured fish, typically laid out on the table when guests arrive, so that those who come early have something to snack on, and those who come later don't feel bad that people have been waiting for them. I usually have a few dishes at a separate table, away from the one where we'll be eating, so that the zakuski table itself is a conversation starter, before even getting to the dining room table.

Next, I love to have a soup course—borscht, or "green borscht," which is traditionally made with sorrel leaves, or potato leek soup, à la Julia Child's recipe. The main course is usually meat or fish with vegetables—classic family dishes and those featuring seasonal foods—and then the final course is dessert and, of course, tea.

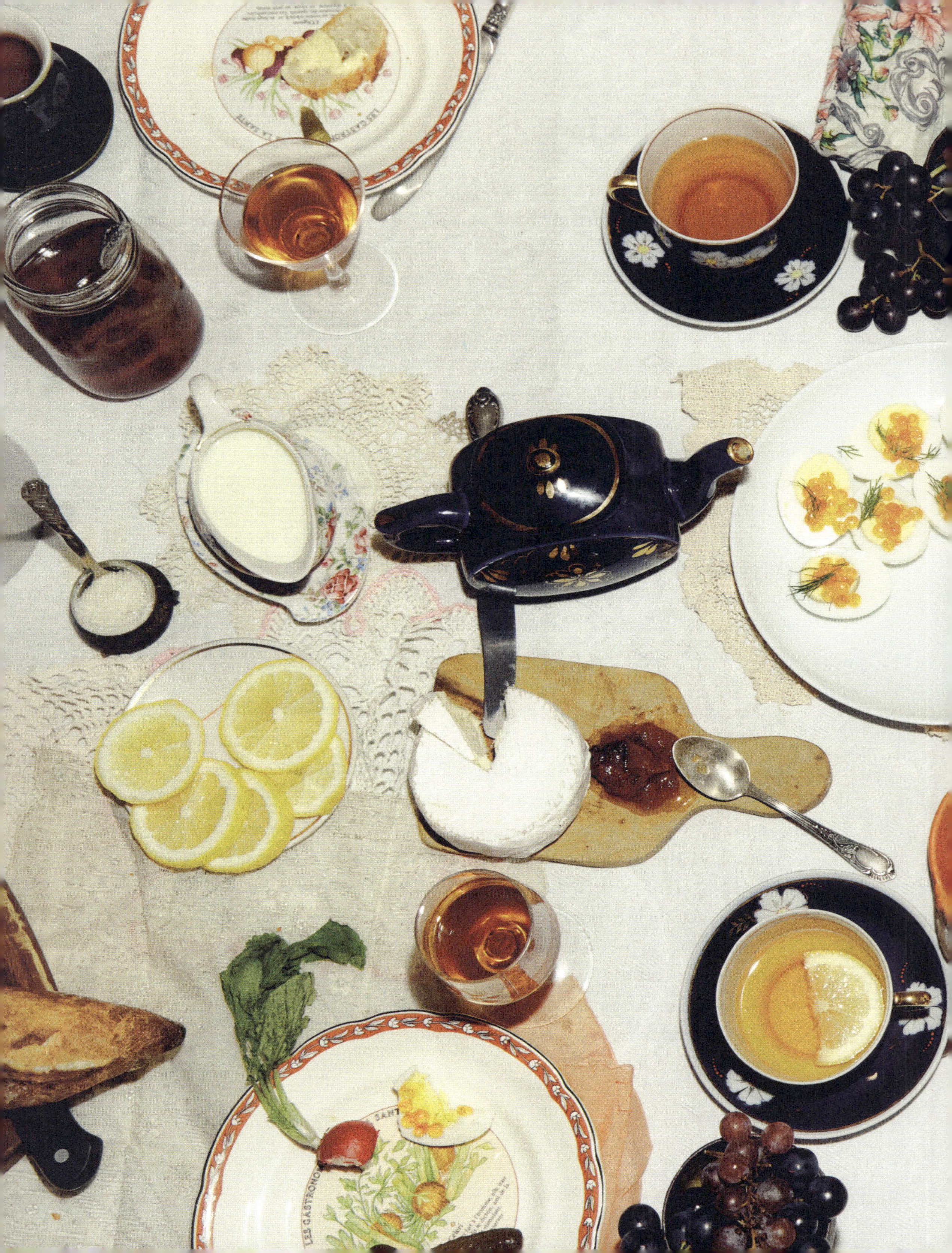

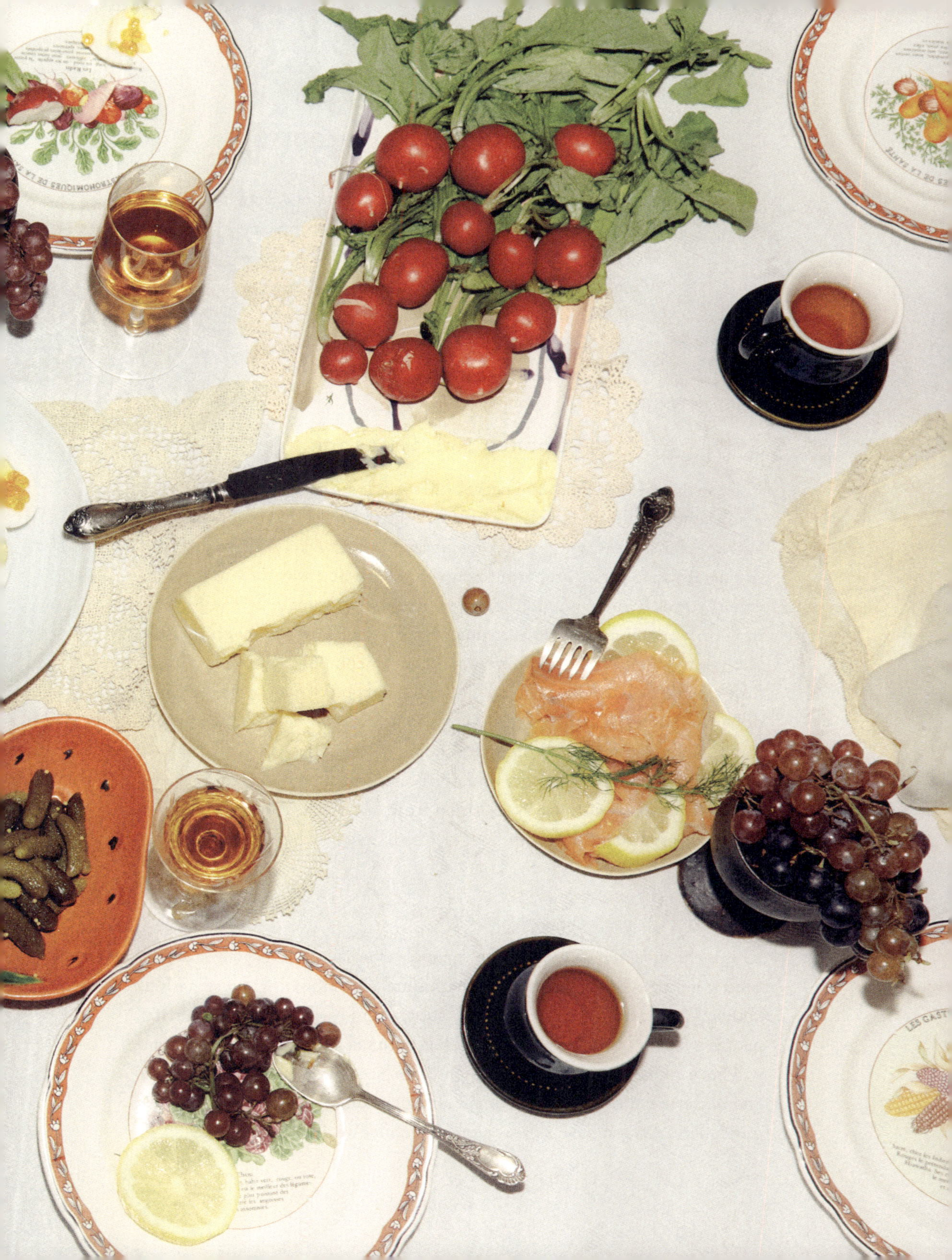

Hosting Smaller Tea Gatherings

"After greetings have been exchanged with guests, they should be honored with fresh tea. After three bowls have been drunk, they should be presented with a bowl of soup of sugarcane, papaya, plums, bayberry, the five flavors, olives, gourds, and winter sunflowers."
—Posthumous edict of Emperor Wu,
Lu Yu, *The Classic of Tea* (780 AD)

A Spontaneous Gathering

You too can be ready for unexpected guests in your home. Like a host with a hot samovar, always have a tea kettle on the stove, ready to fill with water and boil, have a few types of tea on hand, and a small snack like dried fruit or nuts ready to serve. Preparing a cup of tea can be a way for you to easily center yourself and find grounding, while making somebody comfortable in your home. Because you are somewhat distracted in the making of the tea, both you and the guest have a moment to compose yourselves. It's so little trouble to make tea—just boil hot water and pour it over some tea leaves or herbs—but it also denotes care and sharing in a way that a simple glass of water may not (though that of course should also be offered).

Even if you're not hungry and don't have much on hand, bring something out to serve with tea. Nuts, dried fruit, and fresh fruit are best; your guest can have a bite or not, without feeling like they're being rude.

Brunch

This is the most low-key way to have people over for tea: everyone still acts tired from the evening before, has put minimal effort into their presentation, and is the welcoming combination of hungry and easily satisfied. If having people over for brunch, you have to offer both tea and coffee. Many guests will have coffee upon arrival and might have a special cup of tea toward the end of the meal. Even if you yourself are not a coffee drinker, don't be a tea purist here. At least have a French press of coffee available for people.

When it comes to tea at brunch, have the basic options ready: Earl Grey, English Breakfast, Darjeeling black tea. I would have one batch of black tea concentrate (see recipe, page 87) ready so that you can seamlessly make what will probably be most popular. Whereas with dinner I recommend sticking to just a couple of options, with brunch, especially if it's not seated and you're letting guests pick up food and drink for themselves, it can be really fun to have a large variety of tea selections. If you're a baker, a freshly made fruit tart, bread with jam, tea cookies, or cakes work well. Put out what you have! Talk about tea with your guests. Brew individual cups for people based on what they like versus making one or two big teapots for the table. This is especially important because, unlike a dessert course after dinner, people are eating and drinking at different times during a brunch course, so the tea isn't served to everybody at the same time. If you have a way to steam milk at home, make your guests a London Fog, make matcha. This time of day is ideal for making fun, more time-consuming teas for other people. If brunch is in the warmer months, cold brew a couple of iced teas (see recipe, page 94) the night before and serve in beautiful glasses.

Afternoon Tea at Home

If you don't want to cook a full dinner, but still want to host a group, plan afternoon tea. Since tea is the central theme for this, versus food for a brunch or dinner, bring out the best teapots and teacups that you have. For a British-style afternoon tea, you can serve finger sandwiches, scones with jam and cream, and pastries. But if you want to keep it simple, either choose one type of food to make or head to the local bakery in the morning and get an assortment of pastries so you can focus on the presentation rather than the cooking—or serve fresh fruit, crudités, and charcuterie at that hour. The goal of tea at this time is to sit with your guests and engage with them, versus dinner when you might be running to the kitchen to finish up cooking. Have all of your teaware close and select the tea yourself. Green tea can be great at this time because, while it does have caffeine, it's not really enough to keep people awake at night. I like to also have black tea available for those who don't mind the caffeine, because you can serve it with milk, honey, and lemons, which are all ways to beautify the table.

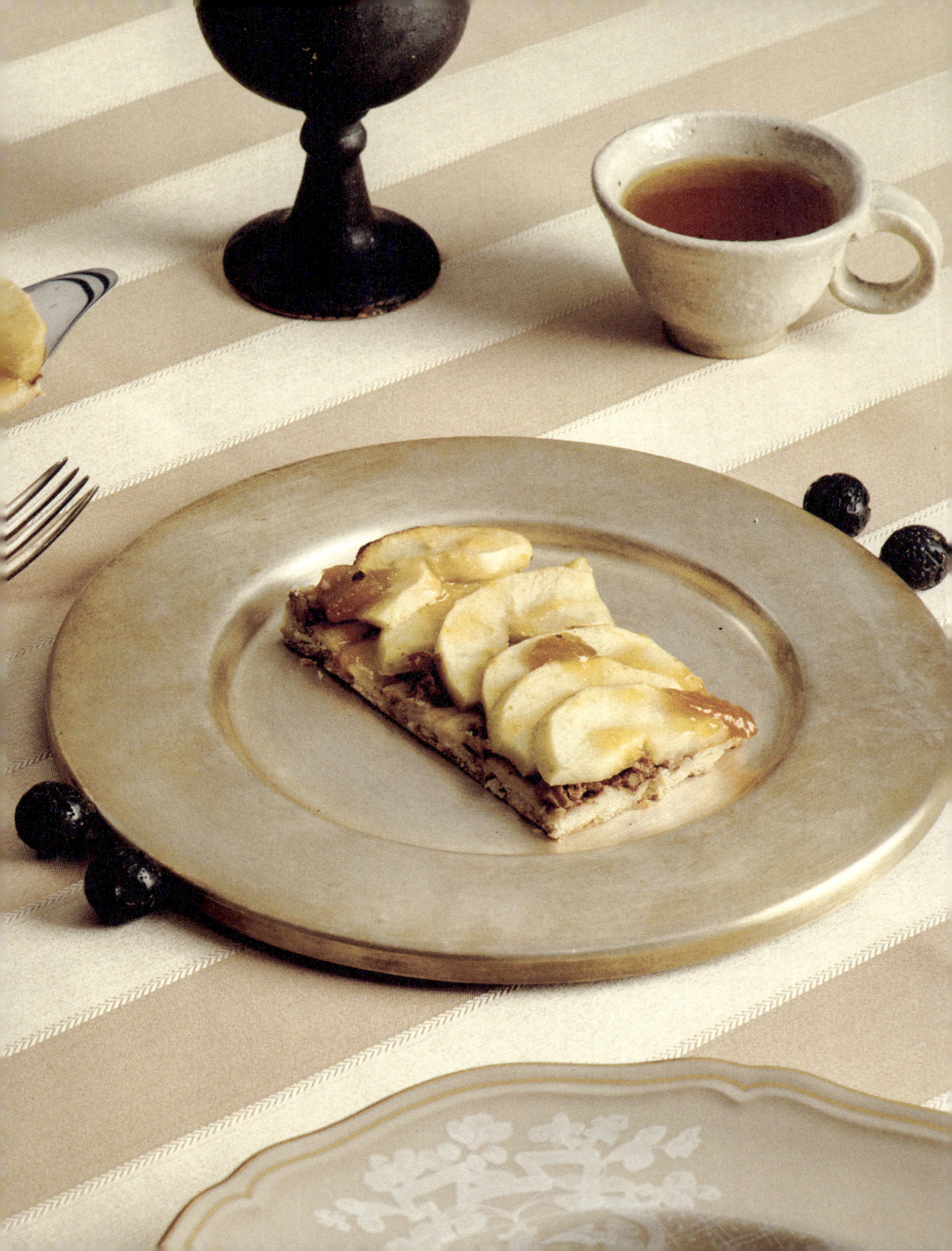

Picnics with Tea

An extension of tea at home is tea at a picnic. I often have picnics with friends and family when the weather is nice. If everyone is bringing something potluck style, consider bringing tea. There are several ways to seamlessly incorporate tea into this tradition. The first and most delightful way is preparing cold brew (see recipe, page 94). If you go to the farmers market the day before, you can incorporate herbs from the market into your cold brew. You can either strain it at home and bring it ready to go, or bring a strainer with you to the picnic. If possible, bring a bag or a thermos full of ice. You can similarly bring hot water in a thermos and prepare hot tea, but for outdoors on a picnic-worthy day, cold brew is easier. Enamel is best for picnics: it is shatterproof and super lightweight, making it easy to transport back and forth, and it works great with cold beverages (it can be hot to the touch with hot drinks). Homemade iced tea elevates a picnic and is also a chic addition to bring as a guest when somebody else is hosting a picnic.

Setting the Table

There are the basic rules of a table setting—the fork on the left, the spoon and knife on the right—and beyond that, in the realm of your own home table, is the fun tablescape that you can create and replicate. For the tea service, you'll need teacups, with or without saucers, and spoons, in case somebody wants honey or sugar. Linen napkins for guests, and also for the tea that inevitably gets spilled on the table, a cute creamer, dessert plates, and both tiny spoons and tiny forks available for cake (ask people their preference). I always offer water alongside tea, sometimes still, sometimes sparkling, in glass cups.

Textiles, Tablecloths, Linens

Cotton, linen, or flax are used for tea towels, tablecloths, and even picnic blankets. Tea towels create opportunity to incorporate color, texture, and patterns to a tea service. I recommend getting several sets of linen napkins with matching tablecloths that are close enough that you can mix and match them with one another. This makes creating a tablescape seamless.

Use tablecloths as a way to alter the space and make it something new. You first of all probably want to protect wooden tables from hot teapots, so that's one reason for their use. But perhaps you want to create a clean, crisp experience, which you can do with a monochrome fabric. If you want to create a more casual lunch vibe, have a gingham or checkered set. Tablecloths are also a great way to temporarily bring new colors into a space. Let's say your dining room is mostly muted colors. If you have a pink tea set, it could be fun to have a pink and green set of linens for the table to match the set. Linens are a noncommittal way to bring in color. Linen fiber is made from flax and it dries faster than cotton, making it suitable for tableware. While I have linen tablecloths that I love, I also have a giant piece of canvas that I use for a tablecloth and have gotten large swaths of fabric from the fabric store in a pinch when wanting to create a specific mood. I think it's okay when tablecloths get the inevitable food and drink stains—just cover those areas with candles or plates or teapots before people sit down.

Silverware

You'll want a set of adorable teaspoons and tiny dessert forks for the dessert and tea course. The spoons for mixing in honey, sugar, or jam, and the forks for whatever desserts or snacks you may serve with a tea. Choose traditional silver, though you'll have the added step of cleaning those with silver cleaner, or simple metal ones. If serving butter or jam, you'll of course need knives for spreading it onto scones or toast.

Other Mood-Setting Elements

Having people over for tea is an intimate form of hospitality and, aside from the tea itself, you can set the mood for a memorable gathering by keeping certain details in mind. I remember going on a date to a teahouse in the East Village and what I remember most from that date, I never saw the person

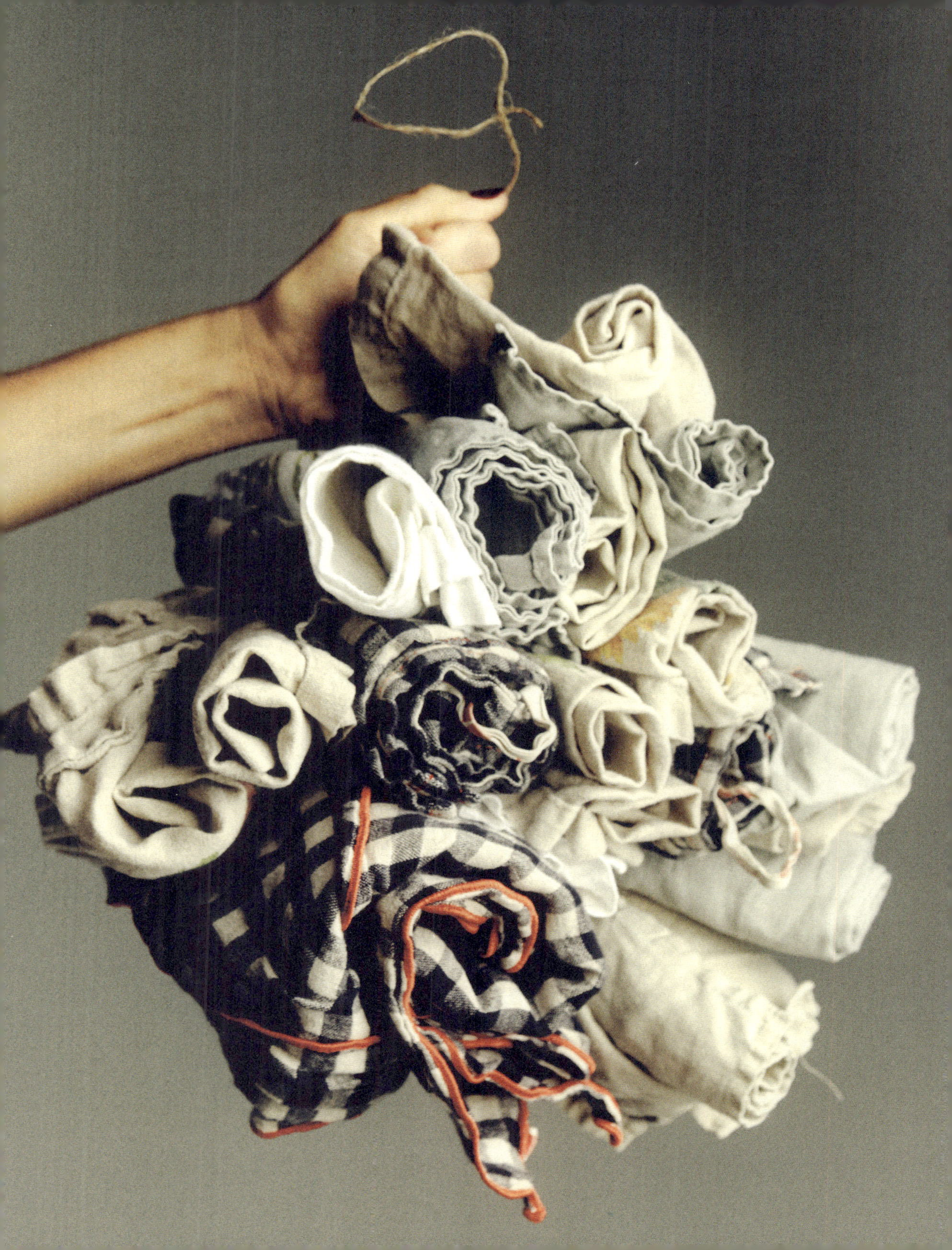

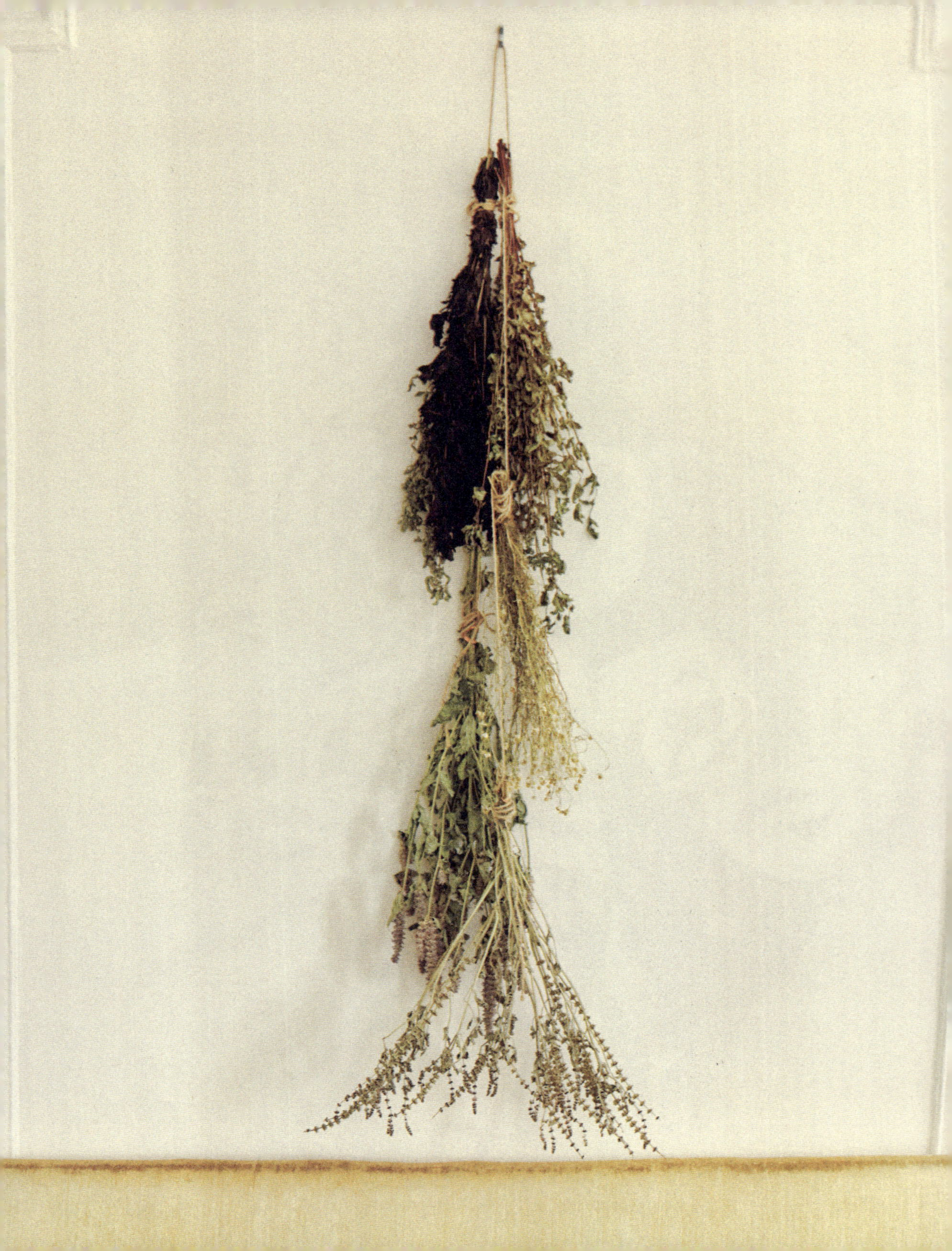

again, was how painfully bright the lights were in the tearoom. At best, a tea party gathering, whether a date or a huge party, should feel effortless, like the decisions you made as the host were naturally correct, rather than considered. And yet, the feeling of effortlessness that a guest takes from a host often comes from a thoughtful sensibility. Below are some of these aspects to keep in mind. Consider lighting, seating, and decorating with flowers—you don't need to incorporate every element, but rather the ones that resonate with you.

Lighting

Natural light, lamps, and candles can all create atmosphere. Tea at home should not be served under harsh lighting. Aggressive, overstimulating lighting is antithetical to teatime. If entertaining in the evening, place candles on the table or around the room. Of course, you can use tealights, but I also love the dramatic effect of beeswax tapers. If you don't have candleholders, a trick I like to use is to cut grapefruits in half, then cut about an inch off the top and bottom so that they'll sit flat on the table, and stick a candle in each grapefruit half, making sure they're secured by pushing the candles in as deeply as possible or dripping some candle wax on the site to "glue" the candles to the grapefruit halves. You can use many other large fruits and vegetables of your choosing as candleholders when you're in a bind. If the room you're having tea in doesn't have much natural light, you can bring candles out even earlier, in the afternoon. If you really, truly don't care and love to hang out under fluorescent lights, at least consider an alternate option if you're hosting guests.

Seating and Setting

People really underestimate the importance of seating. For a large dinner party, seating guests well is the number one, most important thing you can do to ensure success.

FLOOR SEATING: I've always had an area in my home with a coffee table and floor pillows. This setting is so ideal for having tea at home, either by yourself or for a casual gathering with a couple of guests. Sitting on the floor, especially on a rug, can be so cozy and intimate. This isn't comfortable or doable for everybody, so be considerate of guests' abilities if going this route.

AROUND A TABLE: If you're having five or six people over for tea and a meal, people can seat themselves. But if you're having more than six people, it's logistically easier and less awkward for everyone if you arrange seating beforehand. If people are meeting, or are at your house, for the first time, it's gracious to offer suggested seats or, better yet, have place cards on the table. When it comes to seating, put people next to each other who would have something interesting to talk about.

UNCONVENTIONAL SPACES: Japanese architect Terunobu Fujimori designed a series of tea treehouses, accessible by ladder. If there is a way in your home to recreate the magical feel of that kind of a concept, find it and do it. For me, in New York, it's tea on the fire escape. There's only room for myself and one other person, but it can be a really fun experience crawling out the window to sit there. If you have a garden, sitting outside at a table can be similarly transporting. If you have a sauna, creating a tea-table setup for guests to make tea before or after would be another example.

Plants and Flowers

There is an enormous oak tree outside my living room window. On a rainy spring day, I like to watch the wet leaves dance from side to side. On that type of day, I choose to share tea close to that window. In the evening, I might seat guests in the room with all of my books, hopefully with a floral bouquet nearby. The Japanese art of *ikebana*, floral arranging, is a central part of tea ceremony. I shop for flowers at the farmers market, where I can get local, seasonal flowers. The closer to the source you buy the flowers, the lower the impact on the planet and the more supportive you are to your local economy. In the winter, markets will often have dried flowers or branches.

Cleaning Up

Clean up should be done immediately after any party. After a large celebration, having tea with the couple of people who stay behind to help clean while putting things away can lead to the best part: reflection and conversation about the evening. Black tea while cleaning up can provide the small caffeine boost needed to keep going, or something like a chamomile tea can be used to wind down while cleaning.

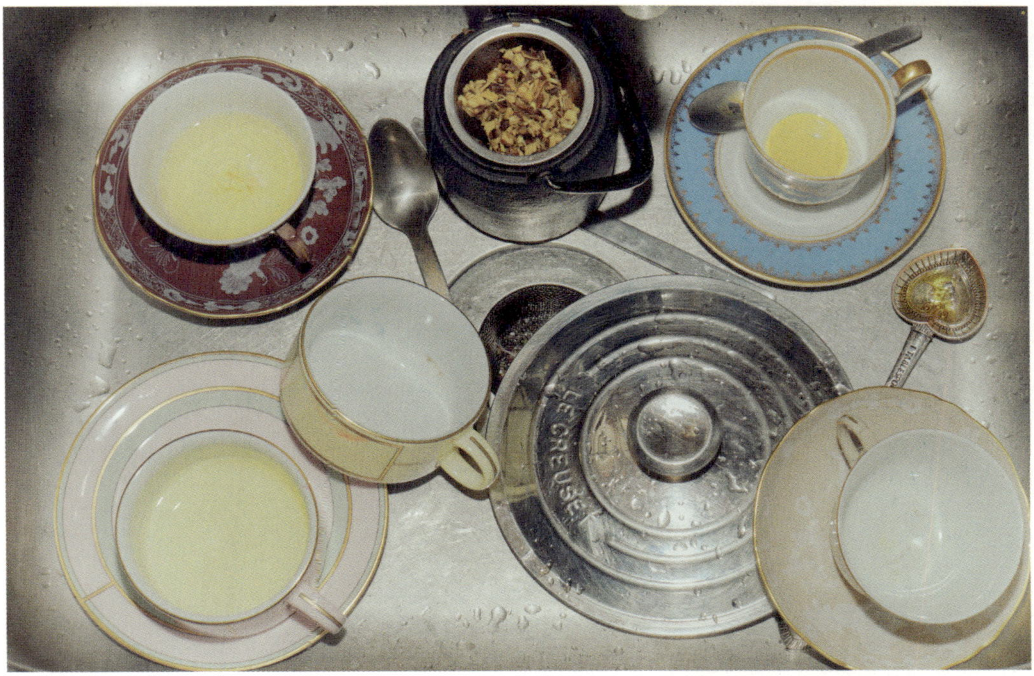

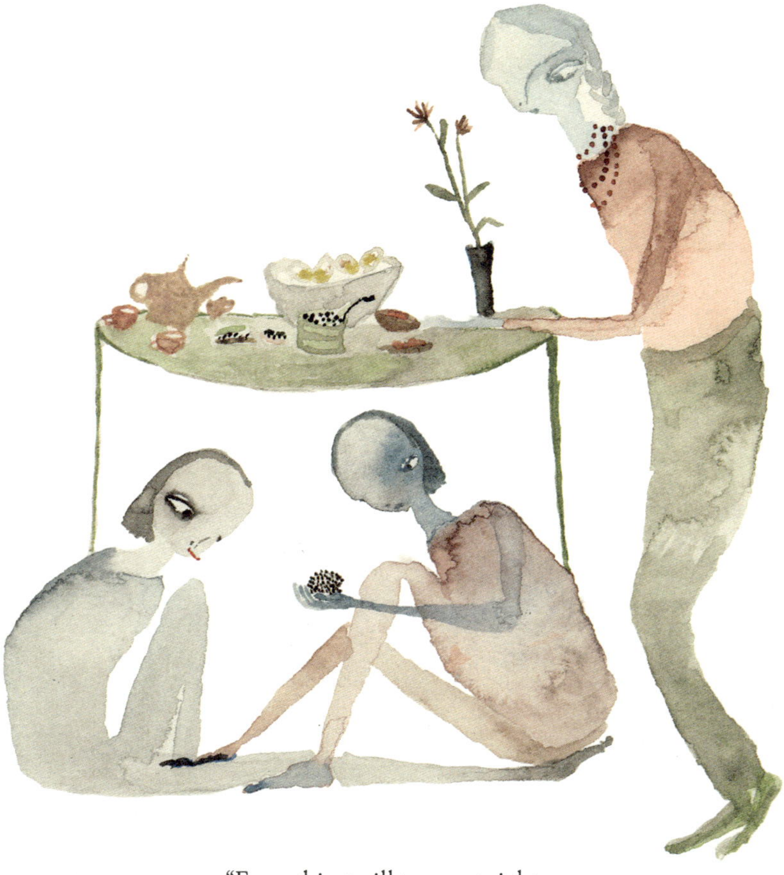

"Everything will turn out right,
the world is built on that."
—Mikhail Bulgakov,
The Master and Margarita (1967)

– 9 –

Babushka Rita's Desserts to Serve with Tea

Though she was born and raised in Kiev, in the USSR, I knew my grandmother, whom I called Babushka Rita, as a New Yorker. She lived in New York City for thirty years, until her death. Whenever I pass Carnegie Hall, or the movie theater near Union Square where she would go every weekend during opera season to watch the opera, live streamed, I think of her New York. I think of her New York when I recreate the recipes in this chapter. These are the desserts I grew up eating at her Brooklyn apartment, on special occasions and ordinary ones alike. "Nobody can live without Brooklyn," my grandmother would always say.

Rita was an excellent host, and, equally important, a great guest. For both of these roles, she had a repertoire of stories, jokes, songs, and five or six pastry recipes that she recycled and that her friends and family would ask and hope for. On the hosting side, her home was always clean, with a display case full of Soviet tea sets, cognac glasses, and even a box of cigarettes in case somebody needed one. She had matching plates and silverware for service, funny stories, a listening ear, and plenty of unsolicited advice. The sensory experience at the table included color and texture through food, but also the emotional spectrum—laughter, war and love stories, probing questions. As a guest, she never came empty-handed, and often delighted everyone at the table by bringing dessert and the skill to make conversation with absolutely anybody, whether she knew them or not.

These recipes are from those times. One day when I went to visit her, my grandmother handed me a Backstreet Boys–themed address book from the nineties in which she had written all of her recipes for me. I have translated and recreated them here.

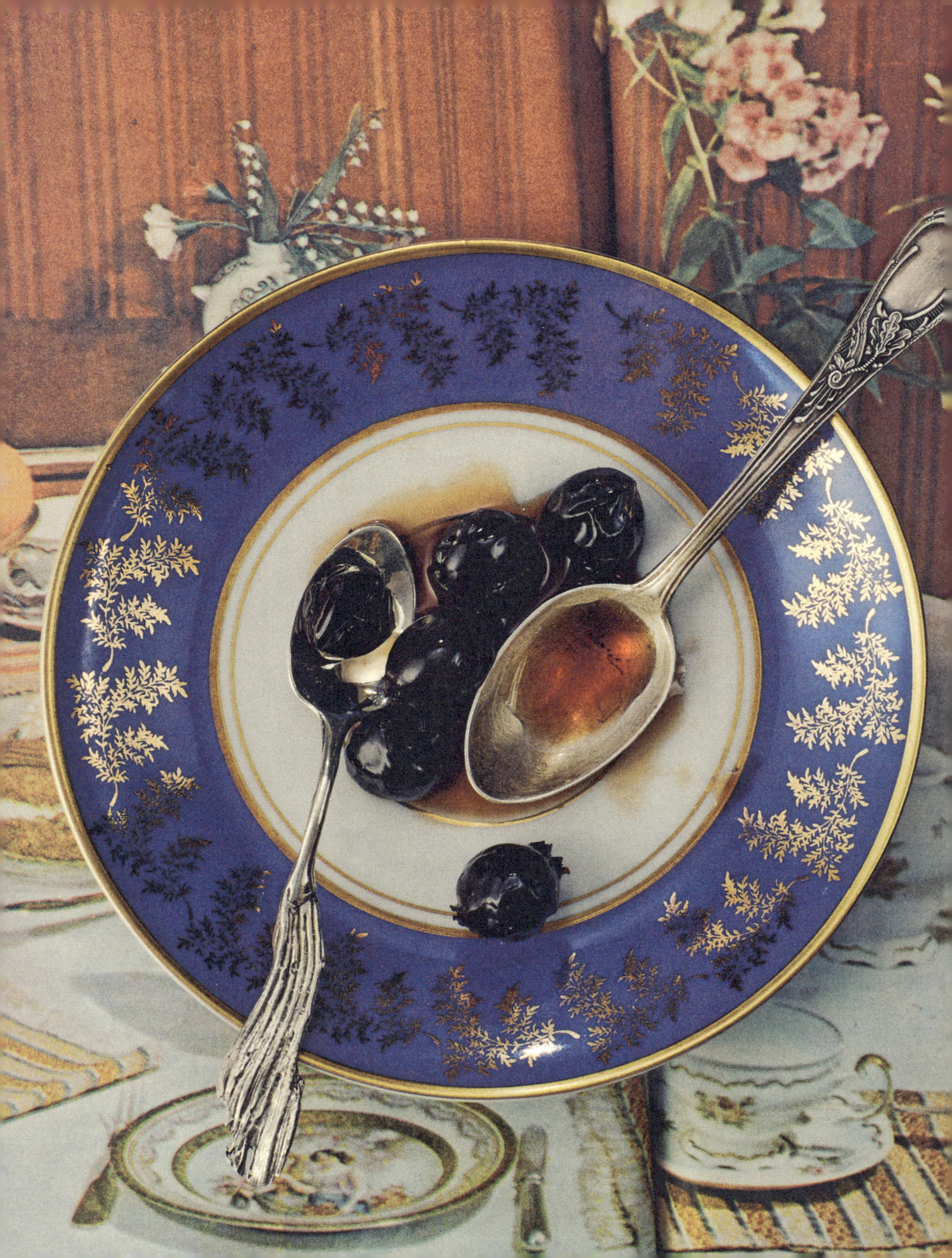

Core Ingredients

This style of baking incorporates some essential ingredients.

FARMER'S CHEESE: It resembles a denser cottage cheese. If you can't get ahold of farmer's cheese, ricotta is a fine substitute in these recipes.

JAM: Apricot, sour cherry, blueberry—jam of any kind is a favorite side to serve with tea. For these recipes, I provide suggested jams to use within them—the ones that my grandmother used—but you can substitute different fruit jams as you see fit.

LEMON: Tea pastries are best with a hint of tartness to balance both the tannins in tea and also the inevitable sweetness of the other pastry ingredients. I buy small, organic lemons. Consider Meyer lemons if you want a more pronounced tartness.

SOUR CHERRIES: Sour cherry season lasts for just a few weeks in the summertime, creating the bright, small, almost pink, tart little fruits. When buying store-bought, remember that sour cherry jam should use whole cherries, rather than being a uniform texture. You'll know that's the case if it says "may contain pits" on the packaging.

SOUR CREAM: Using sour cream in dough creates a density and richness of flavor. I always opt for organic dairy products, favoring local farms, since those are the products that are fresher, without preservatives.

WALNUTS: Most of these recipes incorporate walnuts. In my grandmother's recipes she wrote, "cut each walnut at least six times." I abridged this note to "finely chop" in the recipes that follow, but I include it to give a sense of the way in which my grandmother worked with these raw ingredients. Cutting a walnut six times is such a visceral way to approach food, versus running it through a grinder for speed and ease.

Peach Jam

Makes about 20 ounces
(you can double the recipe if you want more jam)

Though my grandmother most often made jams from the berries she picked herself, this peach jam recipe is the one she wrote down for me, noting that this same concept and recipe can be applied to any kind of fruit.

Make peach jam in the summertime, when the fruit is in season. When choosing peaches for jam, pick fruits that are ripe but firm. They should not squish easily in your hand, but if they are so hard as to be unripe, they won't have much flavor. I prefer to leave the peaches unpeeled. It makes for a richer texture and color. It looks more like a preserve than the uniform jams you find in grocery stores.

Also, I never get involved with the arduous process of canning. This peach jam is meant to be eaten over days and weeks, stored in the fridge.

1 cup (240 ml) water

1 pound (450 g) raw organic cane sugar

3 pounds (1.4 kg) ripe peaches (about 6 medium), halved and pitted

1 or 2 lemons

In a large, wide-bottomed pot, bring the water to a boil over medium-high heat. Add the sugar and cook, stirring continuously, to create a thick paste. It will look like an inordinate amount of sugar, but don't fret! The peaches have so much liquid in them that they will provide plenty of additional liquid for the jam.

Once a paste forms, turn off the heat, add the peaches to the pot, stir them in, and let them soak in the sugar mixture overnight (or for at least 6 hours). You can leave this covered on the stovetop.

The following morning, cook the peaches in the sugar syrup over medium heat, uncovered, for 1½ hours. Keep an eye on the jam and stir frequently with a wooden spoon to prevent it from burning and sticking to the bottom of the pan as the peaches break down.

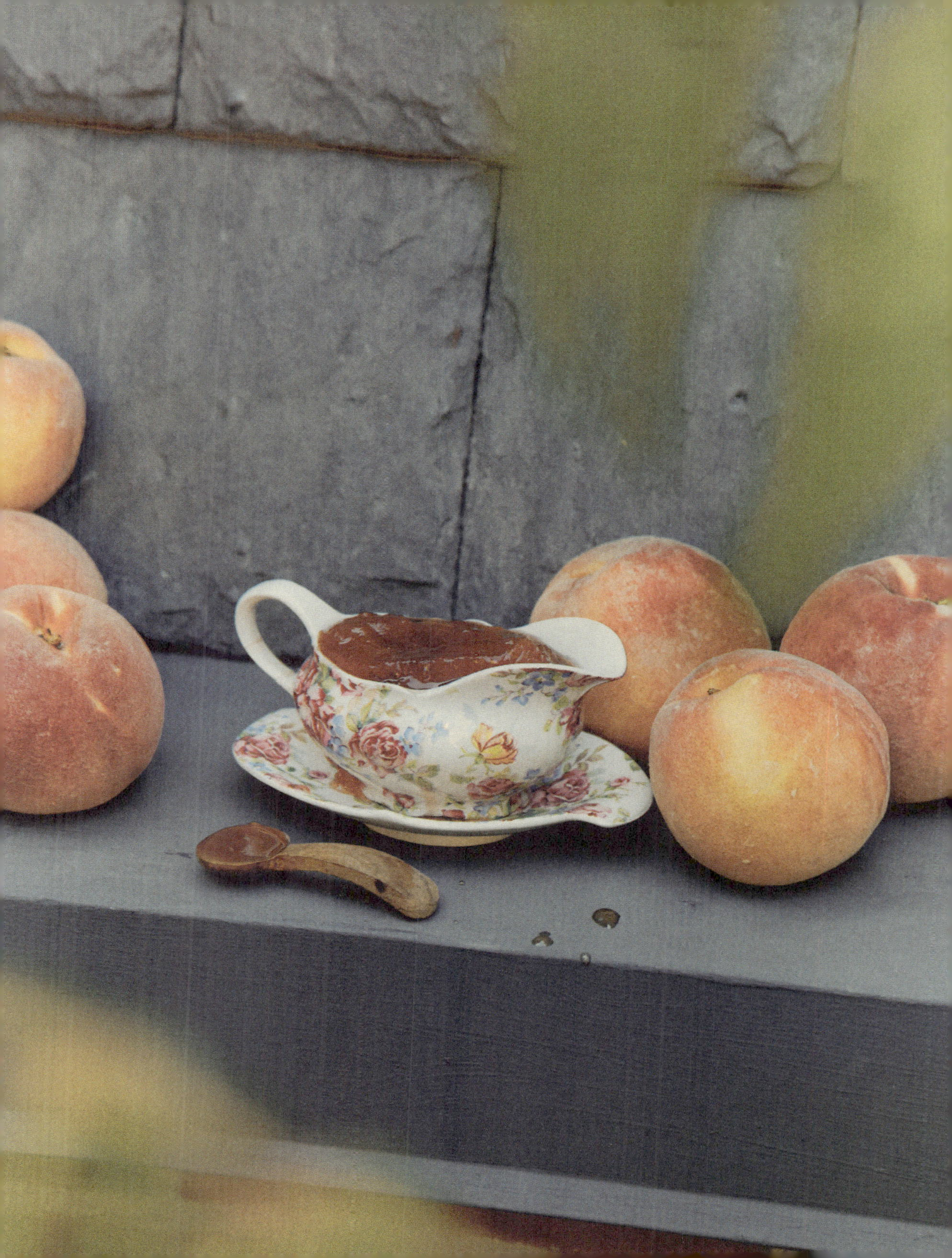

After 1½ hours, add the juice of 1 lemon into the jam and stir it in. If you prefer a more tart jam, you can add the juice of a second lemon. (Avoid store-bought lemon juice as it changes the flavor. If that's all you have, just make it without lemon.)

Continue to cook over medium heat for another 30 minutes to 1 hour (that's 2 to 2½ hours of total cooking time). The jam is done when it looks, for lack of a better word, jammy. This means the peach halves should fall apart when pressed with a wooden spoon (because the peel is left on they will still hold their shape somewhat). You'll also notice that the peaches become translucent and the sugar water turns slightly pink.

Cover the pot and allow the jam to cool for several hours, until it comes to room temperature. The jam will firm up as it cools. To transfer the jam to a glass jar or multiple jars for storage, use a wooden spoon to scoop the peaches into the jars and then use a ladle to pour the cooking liquid over the top. Screw on the lids and refrigerate.

NOTE: After jarring the peaches, you may have leftover liquid. This is great to use for the apple tart recipe in place of apricot jam (page 145).

VARIATIONS: *For a more tart jam,* you can add the zest of 1 lemon when you add the lemon juice. *For a sweeter jam,* use an additional pound of sugar—2 pounds instead of 1 pound.

Sour Cherry Strudel

Makes 12 to 15 servings

Strudel originated in late 1600s Vienna, and became a staple of Jewish cooking. Like the Yiddish language, which my grandparents spoke, recipes from strudel made their way East from Austria, onto Jewish-Ukrainian tables. In my opinion, this sour cherry dessert pairs perfectly with tea: it's not too sweet, it has texture, and the color is moody and sophisticated.

DOUGH

¾ cup (150 g) sour cream

½ cup (115 g) farmer's cheese

1 tablespoon olive oil, plus more for brushing the dough

1 large egg

1 tablespoon water

1½ to 2 cups (180 to 240 g) all-purpose flour, plus more for shaping the dough

FILLING

2 cups (400 g) raisins

1 cup (240 ml) water

1 (8.8-ounce/250 g) jar sour cherry jam

About ½ cup (65 g) breadcrumbs from white, black, or sourdough bread

10 walnuts, finely chopped

Zest and juice of 1 medium lemon (about 3 tablespoons juice)

Ground cinnamon for sprinkling

(recipe continues)

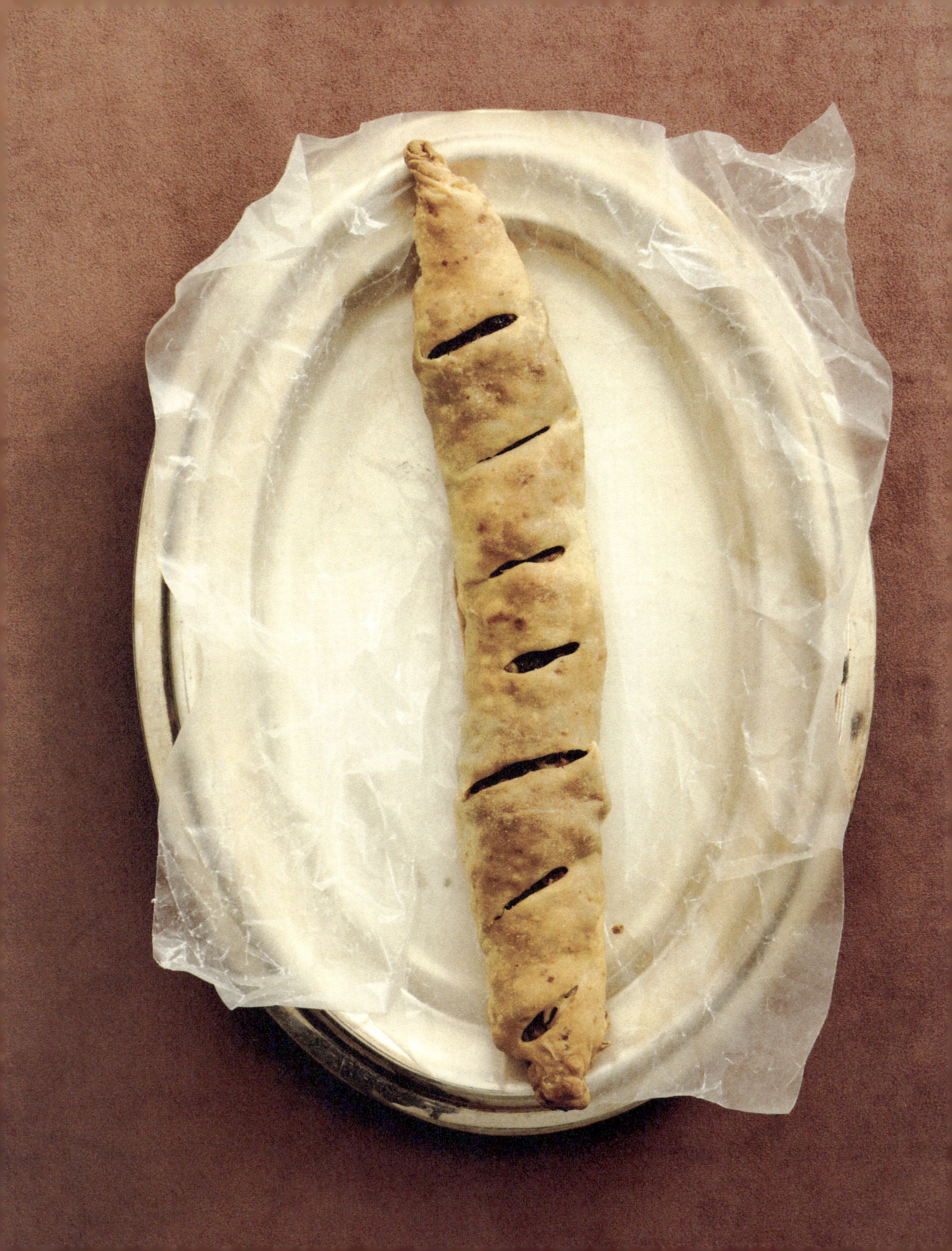

2 tablespoons unsalted butter, melted

Granulated sugar for sprinkling

¾ cup (180 ml) extra-virgin olive oil

MAKE THE DOUGH: In a large bowl, use a wooden spoon to mix the sour cream, farmer's cheese, olive oil, egg, and water until well combined. Add the flour in ¼ cup (30 g) increments and mix it in with your hands as you go; stop adding flour when the dough is still soft but no longer sticks to your hands.

Cover the bowl with plastic wrap and refrigerate for at least 4 hours or up to 3 days.

WHEN YOU'RE READY TO BAKE, PREPARE THE FILLING: Put the raisins and water in a medium saucepan, bring to a boil, then turn off the heat and let sit until you're ready to use them. The water will plump up the raisins.

Using a colander, drain and reserve the liquid from the sour cherry jam. (It's okay to keep a small amount of the liquid in the jam.) Transfer the cherries to a large bowl.

Add about half the breadcrumbs to the cherries, a little at a time, to soak up most of the liquid remaining in the cherries. The breadcrumbs should be soaked, but don't add so many breadcrumbs that the filling completely dries up. Stir in the chopped walnuts.

Using your hands, squeeze all the water from the raisins. Then stir them into the cherry and breadcrumb filling. Add more of the reserved liquid from the sour cherry jam or more breadcrumbs as needed for a just slightly wet mixture. The breadcrumbs should be apparent but the mixture should not be dry. Add the lemon zest and juice.

After the dough has rested in the fridge for at least 4 hours, transfer it to a work surface and separate it into 4 equal pieces. Preheat the oven to 350°F (175°C) while you shape the strudels. Place parchment paper on 1 or 2 large baking sheets.

Flour a work surface and, working with one piece of dough at a time, roll out the dough into a very flat, thin rectangle about the size of a standard sheet of letter paper (8½ x 11 in/ 22 x 28 cm). Brush a thin layer of olive oil on the dough and sprinkle with cinnamon. Spread one-fourth of the sour cherry filling evenly on top.

With one of the longer sides of the dough positioned near you, roll up the dough and seal the edges to enclose the filling. Place the strudel seam side down on a prepared baking sheet. Use a paring knife to make marks about every 2 inches (5 cm) down the roll where you will later cut it. Brush with some of the melted butter and sprinkle with sugar.

Repeat with the three remaining pieces of dough and filling, brushing the tops with the remaining melted butter and sprinkling with sugar. Each of the four long rolls should sit side by side, with about an inch between them. If you need to use two baking sheets with two pieces on each, that's fine. Pour the olive oil over the strudels to coat and brush evenly over the top. Some of the oil will pool on the bottom of the baking sheet, which will serve to lightly fry the pastry.

Bake the strudels for 45 minutes, periodically basting with the pooled olive oil on the bottom of the pan. Remove from the oven when the pastry starts to brown to prevent the strudels from drying out.

Let the strudels rest on a wire rack for at least 20 minutes before serving. Slice the strudels using the marks as a guide and serve warm or at room termperature. Leftover strudel stores well in the fridge in an airtight container for up to 3 days.

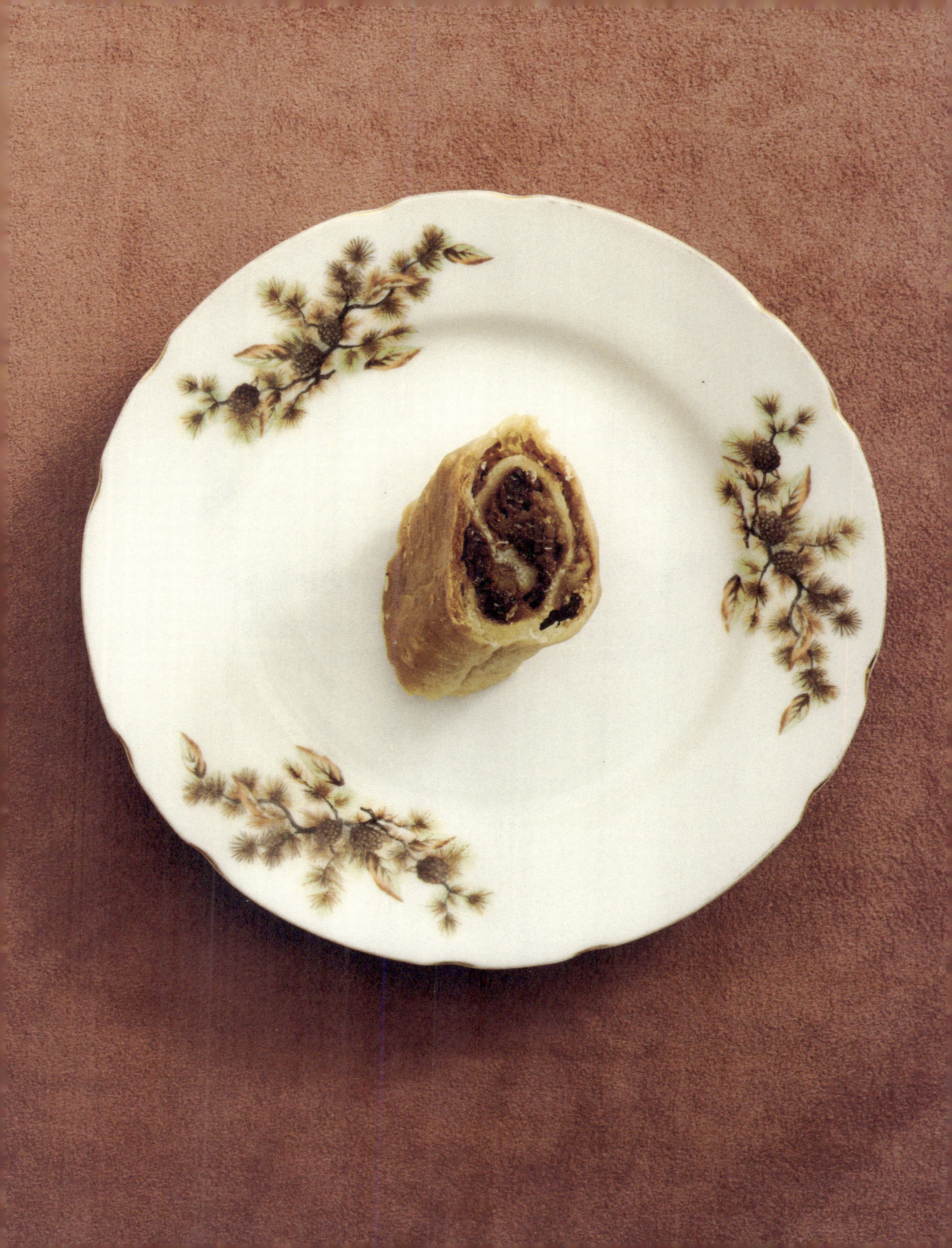

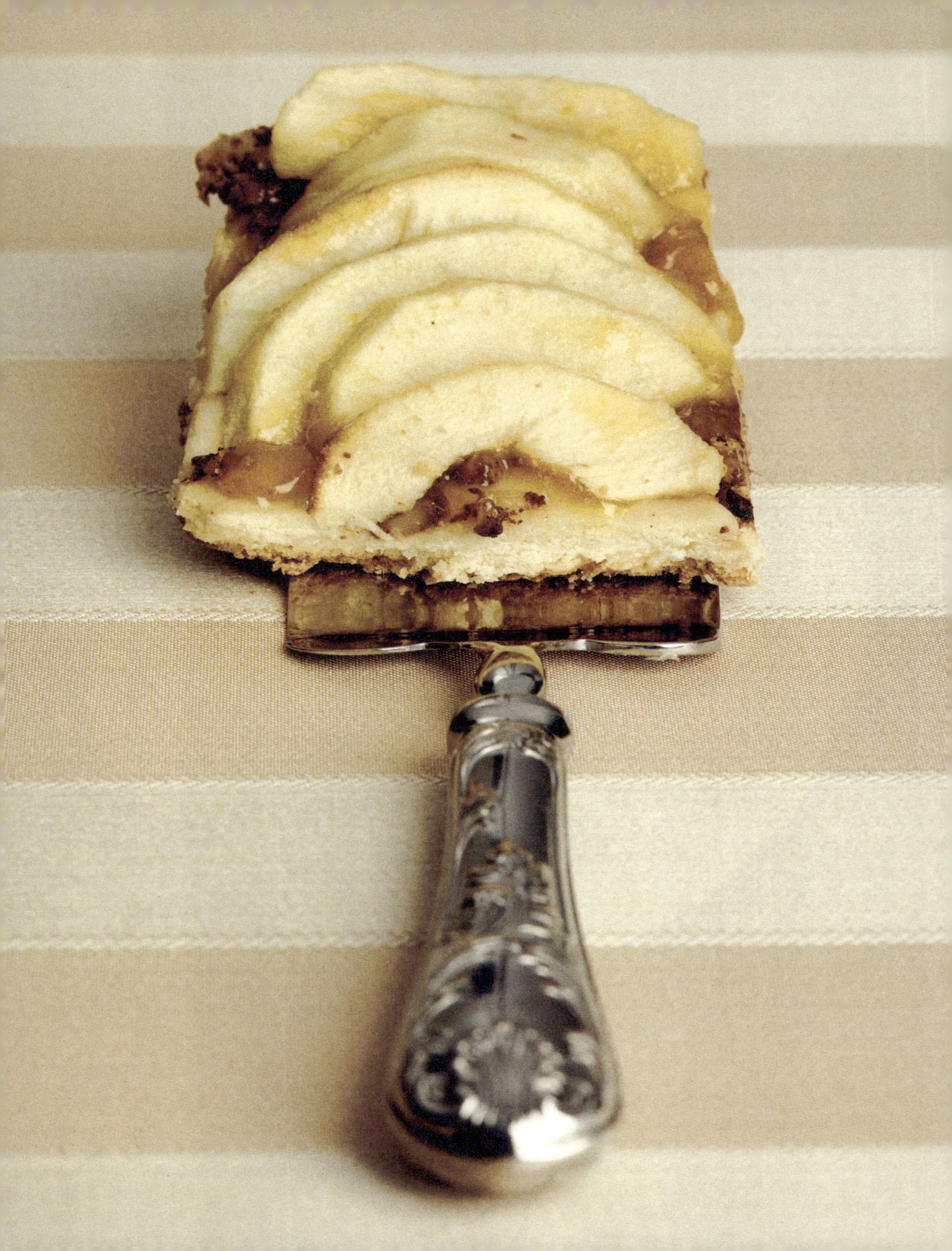

Apple Tart

Serves 12 to 15

My grandmother supposedly adapted this open-faced apple tart from the German fashion magazine *Burda*, which was the first Western magazine to be translated into Russian and distributed in the Soviet Union. She also used the base of this tart to make an American flag tart every Fourth of July (instead of using the nuts and apples for filling, she would cover the tart with cream and then create stripes and stars out of cut strawberries and blueberries). So feel free to adjust this tart recipe to express whatever you need on the top.

DOUGH

2¼ cups (275 g) all-purpose flour

½ cup (100 g) powdered sugar

10 tablespoons (150 g) unsalted butter, softened

1 large egg

2 tablespoons sour cream

FILLING

2 pounds 3 ounces (1 kg) apples
(4 to 5 medium; see Notes)

Zest and juice of 1 lemon (about 3 tablespoons juice)

¾ cup (50 g) walnuts

1 teaspoon ground cinnamon

2 teaspoons (10 ml) vanilla extract

Pinch ground cloves

+ + +

(recipe continues)

½ cup (120 ml) apricot or peach jam, or orange marmalade, warmed on the stovetop (see Notes)

¼ cup (60 ml) cognac

Vanilla ice cream or whipped cream (optional), for serving

MAKE THE DOUGH: Sift the flour into a bowl. Add the powdered sugar, butter, egg, and sour cream. Knead until the dough comes together and roll into a ball. Wrap the dough in plastic wrap and let the dough chill for at least 2 hours in the fridge.

MEANWHILE, MAKE THE FILLING: Peel the apples, cut them into thin slices, and place them in a bowl. Pour the lemon juice over them and stir to coat the apples (reserve the lemon zest for the nuts). Cover the bowl with plastic wrap and refrigerate the apples while the dough finishes chilling.

Run a rolling pin over the walnuts until they are broken up into small pieces. In a small bowl, toss the walnut pieces with the cinnamon, vanilla, ground cloves, and lemon zest. (You can use a whole vanilla bean in place of vanilla extract, just cut the bean in the half and scoop the insides directly into the nut mixture.)

After the dough is chilled, preheat the oven to 350°F (175°C). Roll the dough into a rectangle, about 15 x 10 in (38 x 25 cm) and about ½-inch (1 cm) thick. It may be difficult to roll the dough right out of the fridge, so either let the dough sit on the counter for 15 minutes or work it with your hands to warm it, then wind it around a rolling pin and lay it out on a baking sheet lined with parchment paper. Prick the dough in many places with a fork.

Sprinkle the surface of the dough evenly with the walnut mixture. Place the apple slices on top in overlapping rows, as tightly as possible, with just ½ inch (1 cm) of each apple slice showing underneath the next.

Bake until the edges of the crust start to brown, about 35 minutes.

Remove from the oven. While the apple tart is still warm, carefully spread a thin layer of the warm apricot jam on top, then flambé the cognac over the tart. You can do this by pouring the cognac into a ladle and carefully lighting the cognac with a match, then pouring the cognac generously and evenly over the tart. (Alternatively, if you don't want to flambé the cognac, you can warm it together with the apricot jam and spread the mixture on the tart.)

Before serving the tart, trim off the bare edges of the pastry crust, taking care not to cut into the apples on top. You can serve this tart hot or at room temperature and it's great with vanilla ice cream or whipped cream. It also stores well in the fridge for several days.

NOTES: I love making this tart in the fall with apples from the farmers market. When sourcing apples from your market, ask the farmers what apples they like to use for tarts and pies. They may sell interesting varieties you haven't tried before. I have made this with Honeycrisp, for their texture, and for those who love the most tart apples possible, try Granny Smiths. It's important to choose crisp, fresh apples.

Try to use mostly the liquid part of the jam versus the pieces of fruit, whether apricots or peaches, when making the tart, because the peaches are a little too big and may overpower the apples.

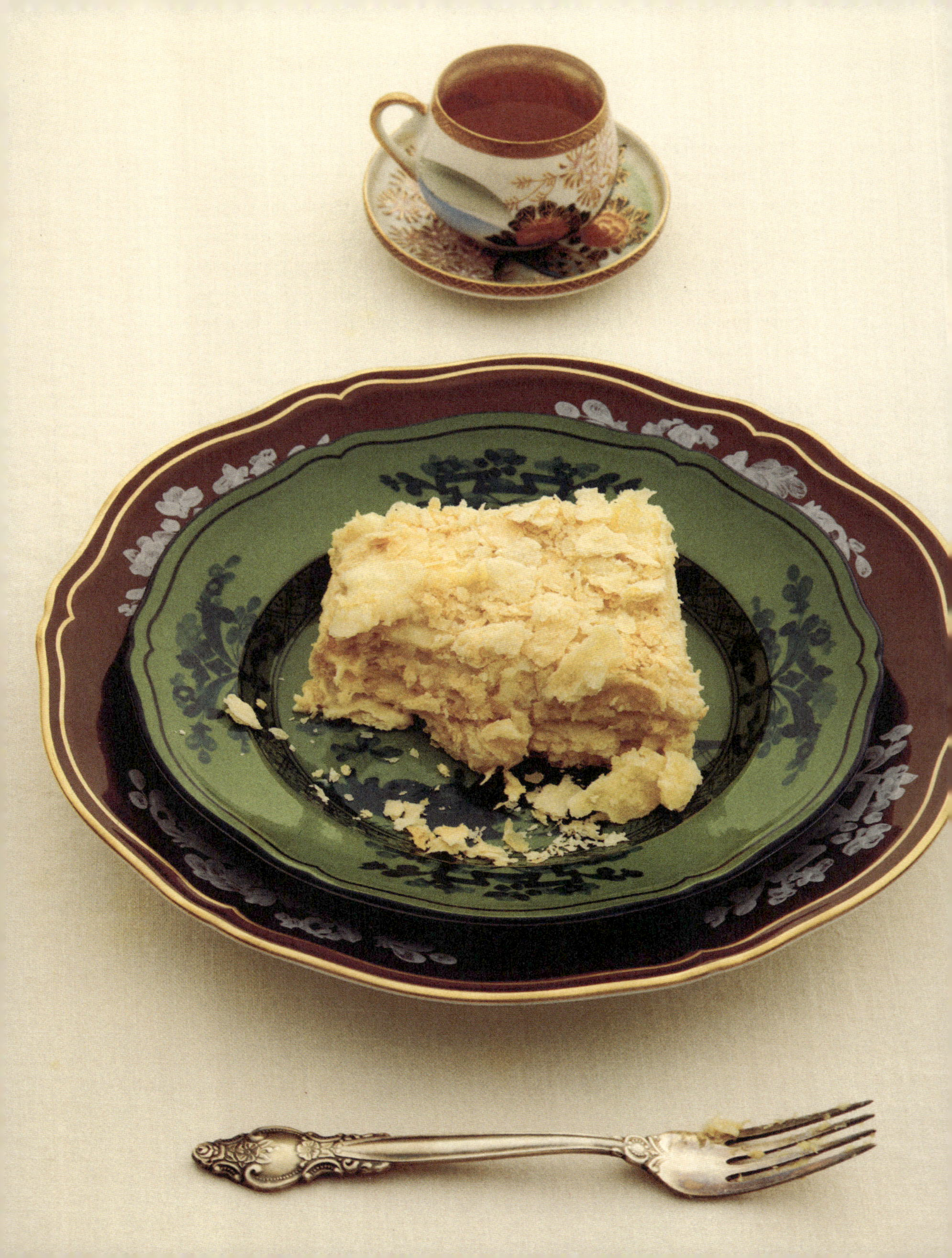

Napoleon

Serves 12 to 15

Inspired by the French mille-feuille pastry, this multilayered flaky pastry was created in Russia in 1912 and so called to celebrate the one hundred years of Russia's victory over France after the Patriotic War of 1812 (which was a disaster for Napoleon). The layer of crumbs on top references the snow in Russia that helped Russian troops defeat the invading French troops during a harsh winter.

This cake is a Soviet staple and versions are found in Russian grocery stores, on New Year's Eve tables, and at celebrations of all kinds. It's made by layering pastry dough with cream. In my grandmother's version, the cream is not cooked on the stovetop but is a simpler blend that incorporates sweetened condensed milk, creating a dense, particular flavor.

PASTRY

14 tablespoons (190 g) unsalted butter, chilled

2 cups (250 g) all-purpose flour, plus more for working dough

⅓ cup (100 ml) cold water

1 egg yolk

Juice of ½ lemon (about 4 teaspoons)

½ teaspoon fine salt

PASTRY CREAM

12 tablespoons (180 g) unsalted butter, softened

1¼ cups (400 g) sweetened condensed milk

2 teaspoons vanilla extract

(recipe continues)

MAKE THE PASTRY: Grate the cold butter on the coarse side of a grater into a large bowl.

Add the flour and use your hands to rub the butter into the flour until you have fine crumbs. Make a well in the center.

In a separate small bowl, whisk the water, egg yolk, lemon juice, and salt. Pour into the well.

Using your hands, knead the yolk mixture into the butter-and-flour crumbs until thoroughly combined and an even consistency. It will take several minutes. Roll the dough to create a ball and wrap in plastic wrap. Refrigerate for at least 1 hour to chill.

Divide the dough into 8 equal pieces and roll each into small balls. Place a large baking sheet in the oven and preheat to 350°F (175°C).

Sprinkle a work surface with flour and use a rolling pin to roll out 1 ball into a rectangle as thin as you can make it without it tearing, about 8 x 10 inches (20 x 25 cm).

Remove the hot baking sheet from the oven and carefully transfer the rectangle to the baking sheet. While the first layer of pastry is baking, roll out the second layer to the same dimensions. Remove the first layer of pastry to a cooling rack when it is lightly brown, about 8 minutes. Set aside to cool (it's okay to stack the pastry sheets while they cool). Repeat with the remaining layers of pastry.

MAKE THE PASTRY CREAM: In a large bowl, beat the softened butter with a handheld mixer until fluffy, which will take several minutes. Whisk in the condensed milk and vanilla extract.

To assemble the cake, place a pastry layer on a serving plate and, using a large knife or the back of a spoon, spread a layer of cream over it evenly. Cover with a second layer and continue until all the cake layers are used except one.

Chop the last layer and any other scraps of cooked pastry into crumbs and sprinkle the top with the crumbs. Cut the edges off so that the final product is an even rectangle.

Refrigerate, covered with aluminum foil or in an airtight container, for at least 6 hours or overnight.

To serve, cut into small pieces. Serve cool or at room temperature.

Catskill Mountain Cake

Serves 8

Originally, my grandmother called this Tort Carpath, after the Carpathian Mountains in Central Europe, but after moving to New York City and spending summers in the Catskills, she renamed it to reflect the new mountains that were her summer home. The Catskill Mountains in upstate New York are actually the oldest mountain range in the country, and I think the name is lovely for this no-bake mountain-range-shaped cake.

You could theoretically make rectangular shaped tea cookies at home in place of store-bought, but my grandmother created this recipe using things that she already had lying around at home, and so this cake was made in that spirit.

1 tablespoon (9 g) black tea leaves (or 3 tea bags)

1 cup (240 ml) hot water

1 cup (225 g) farmer's cheese

½ cup (115 g) sour cream

1 tablespoon honey

2 tablespoons finely chopped walnuts (optional)

2 teaspoons cacao powder

2 tablespoons sour cherry jam

36 tea biscuits, preferable Kedem,
plus more for base (optional)

Powdered sugar for dusting

Chocolate syrup (optional)

Make a strong hot black tea by placing the tea leaves in a large mug and pouring the hot water over them. Let it brew until it comes to room temperature (you can brew the tea the night before or a few hours before you plan to make the cake).

(recipe continues)

In a medium bowl, mix the farmer's cheese, sour cream, honey, and walnuts, if using. Divide this mixture into thirds and place in three separate bowls.

Leave the contents of one as is, mix the cacao into the second bowl, and sour cherry jam into the third. (Or you can also do just sour cherry filling or just chocolate filling or whatever combination you choose; you don't have to use three different flavor/color profiles.)

Lay a sheet of aluminum foil (at least 10 x 12 inches/25 x 30 cm) on a work surface.

Quickly dip an entire biscuit in the tea—it only needs to be in the tea for a second—and place down, facing you. For the first layer, you will use 12 cookies to make a 4 x 3 grid (4 rows of 3 cookies each).

Spread the plain mixture over the biscuits using a butter knife or the back of a spoon.

Continue with dipping 12 biscuits into the tea and create another grid of 12 cookies on top of the cream layer. Cover with the cacao mixture.

Continue dipping another 12 biscuits in tea and laying them down on top of the cacao layer for your third and final layer. Spread this layer with the sour cherry mixture.

From the longer, horizontal sides (where there are four cookies, versus the shorter vertical sides with three cookies) bring the foil upward to make a triangle (mountain peak) shape. The foil will hold it in place and mold it into shape.

Refrigerate the cake overnight, or for at least 6 hours, before serving. This is best served cold so it maintains its shape. Right before serving, remove the foil and consider sprinkling the top with powdered sugar or pouring chocolate syrup over it—it will look slightly uneven from being covered in aluminum foil. When it's cold, it's easy to transfer and maintains its shape well. You may present it to your guests on a serving platter or over a base of cookies (optional; pictured). If presenting it on a cookie base, bring it back to the kitchen after you've shown it off to cut it into 1-inch slices and plate it.

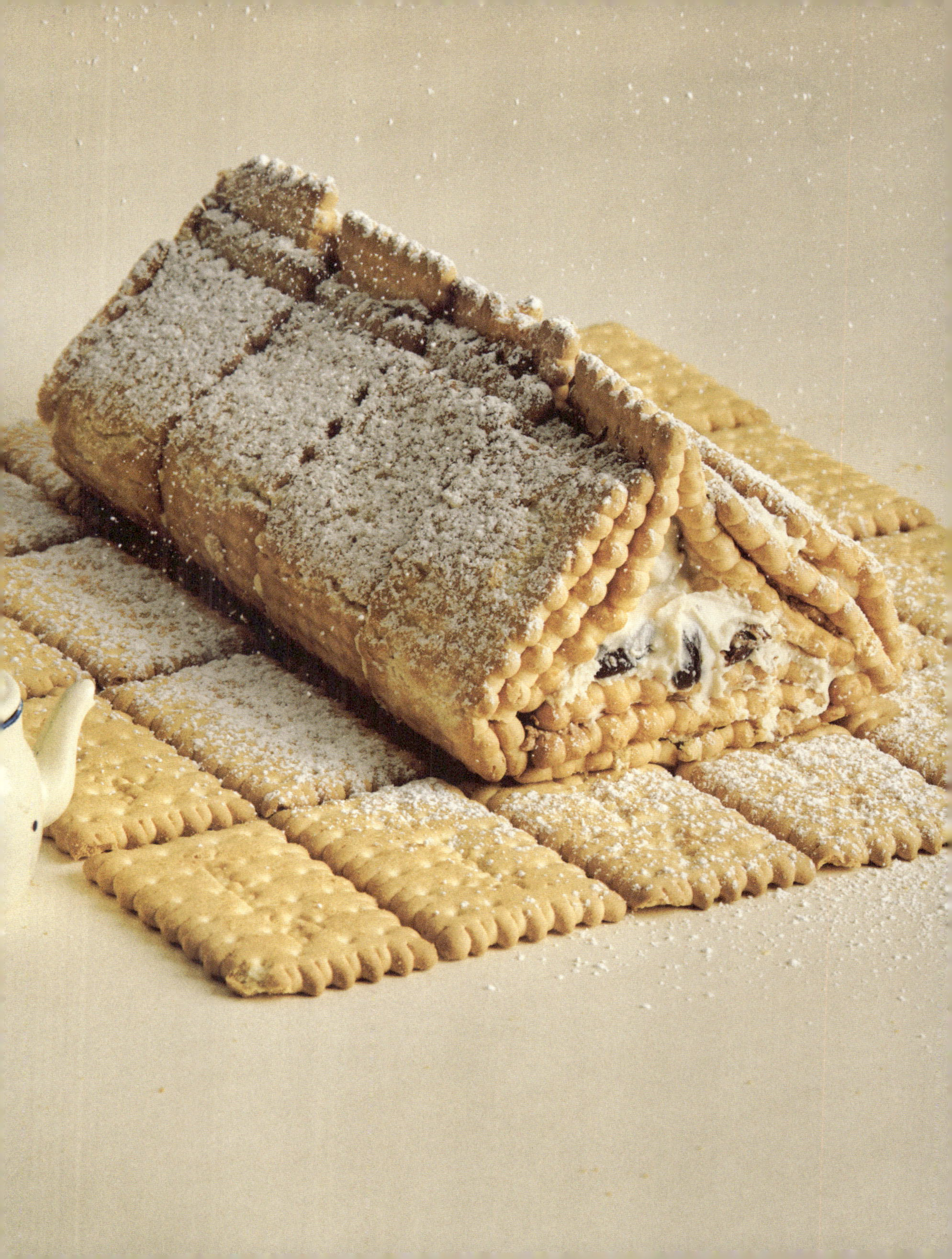

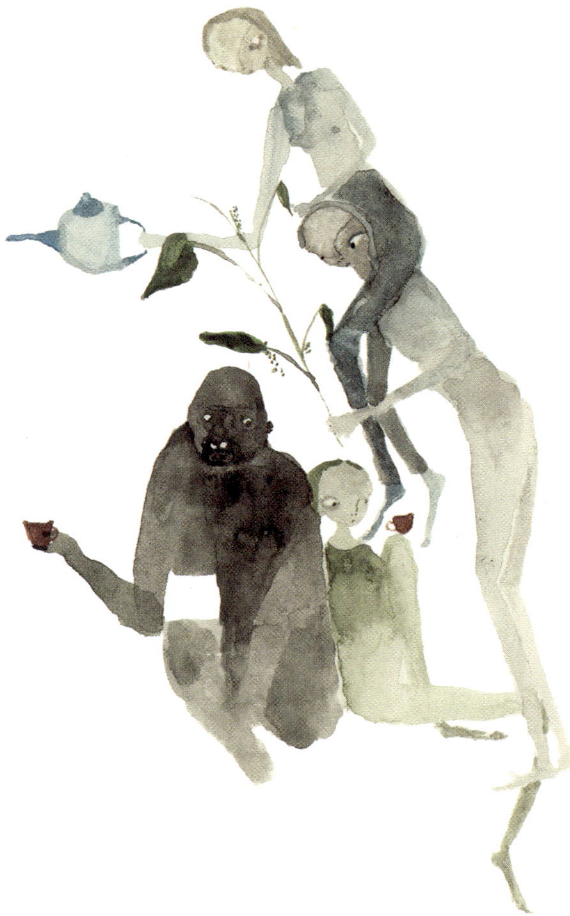

"Would you like an adventure now,
or shall we have our tea first?"
—J. M. Barrie, *Peter Pan* (1902)

– 10 –

Tea with Children

Something that surprised me after having a child is how often tea imagery arises in classic children's books. Peter Rabbit's mom is always making chamomile tea and Mother Goose rhymes about it.

Polly put the kettle on, Polly put the kettle on,
Polly put the kettle on, we'll all have tea.

Frog and Toad are constantly drinking tea, Angelina Ballerina's mom loves to serve it. Of course, there's Alice in Wonderland and a favorite Japanese bear, Kuma-Kuma Chan, who makes "bear tea." Many children's book authors continue to incorporate teapots and tea drinking into their stories. Perhaps it's because tea is multisensorial and so innately wonderful for children. There are the colors and shapes of the teapots, the smell of tea leaves, the color of the brewed tea, the taste of accompanying sweets, whether in the form of honey in the tea or of cookies alongside. There's the communal element, making imaginary tea for the child's toys and stuffed animals, or sharing actual tea with friends and parents. Then there is the cozy element of being cared for, of a mother making tea for a child when they are sick. There is also the added element of play sophistication—of dressing up and having an imaginary tea party with miniature toy tea sets, of playing a grown-up in the world.

Tea with children can be fun and exciting: They get to use pretty cups and choose flavors and do the things that the characters in their favorite books do. It can be a way to expand their palates from an early age, it can be a tool to teach sharing through serving tea to one another, and it can be a way to give them a dose of calming herbs before bedtime.

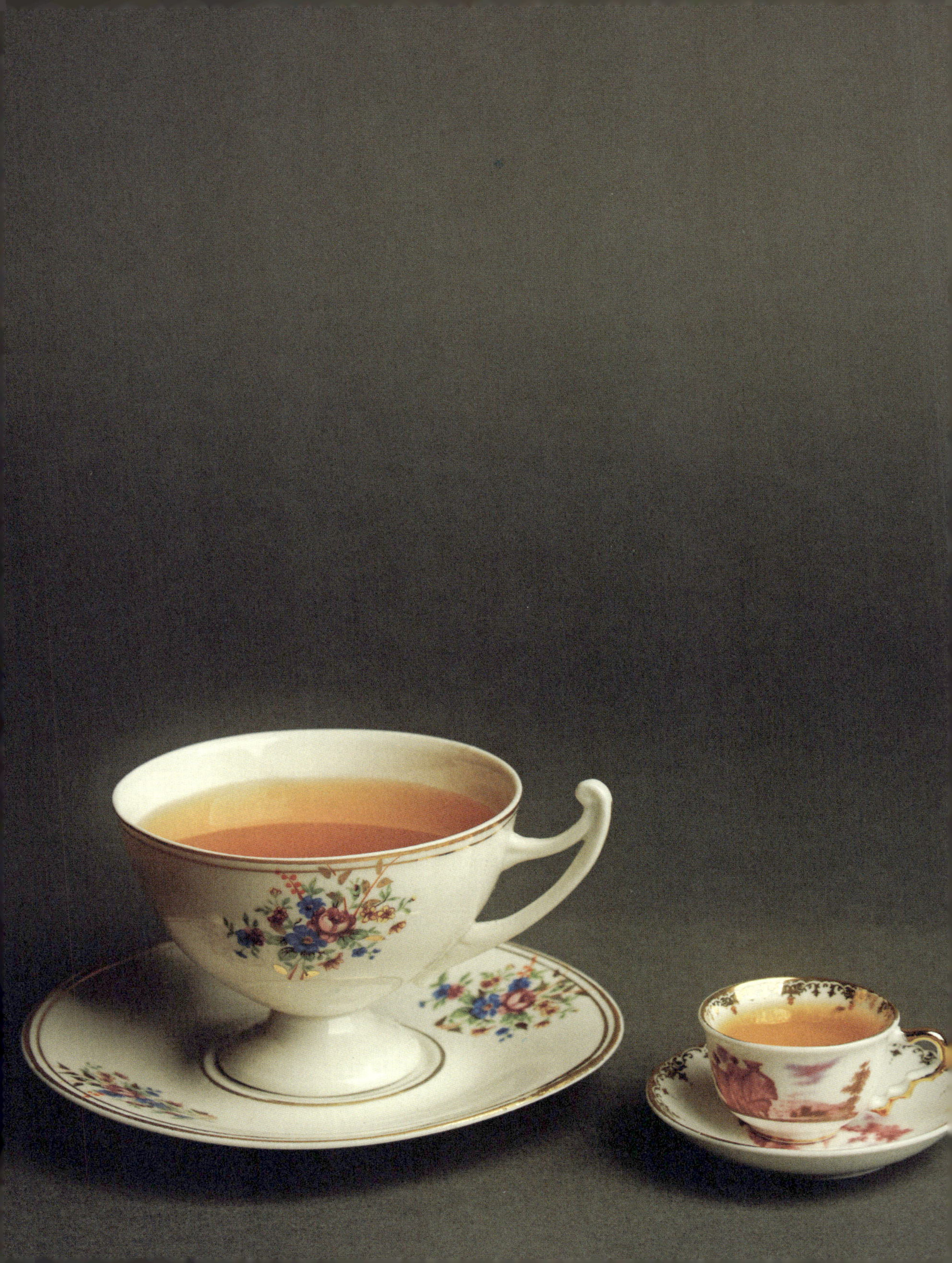

How to Throw a Tea Party for Kids

I threw my daughter, Mona, a tea party for her third birthday. We made a little library of tea-themed books and had toy tea sets for the kids to play with. Whether throwing a small gathering or a large birthday party, bring in elements of different kinds of play for kids of different interests, abilities, and ages. Make a coloring corner with images of teacups and pots (I drew my own and made copies of them), create a photo corner with enamel teapots as props. Multitier stands for afternoon tea are adorable when filled with cupcakes or tiny cookies. Along with serving tea, you can serve milk, water, or juice in tiny teacups. Add in an option for dressing up—there is nothing cuter than a bunch of toddlers in dresses and suspenders.

Choosing Tea for Children

When my daughter was around one, I left a half-finished ceramic bowl of holy basil tea out on the coffee table. I looked up and there she was, holding the bowl with both hands, pouring the tea into her mouth, with most of it landing on her adorable belly, smiling between every sip. Having Mona instinctively enjoy it the same way that I do was the sweetest thing and speaks to the universality of an herbal experience. It also makes me wonder how much of our developed tastes come from what we're exposed to as little ones and how much is just innate preference.

For children, it's best to keep to single flavors, so that you can understand what your child likes: chamomile, mint, and lemon balm are great. Though I started drinking (caffeinated) black tea with milk at a very young age, there are a plethora of herbal options, and I would recommend waiting to introduce caffeine until the teenage years.

When it comes to kids, one way to interest them in teas that they're drinking and the ones that you are, is to make teas of different colors and to bring them into conversations around these teas.

As much as possible, share your tastes starting when they are little. If a tea you make is not well received, then have backup options, but your tastes (in tea and otherwise) are the best starting point. Maybe your own tastes will change in the process.

Mona has picked up many herbal teas. I brought home tiny, precious ceramic cups from Japan and a bag of tea from a small Japanese village with the only English on the package identifying it as "Wild Herb Tea." I made a pot of it for me and my husband, and Mona insisted on a cup. Risking her dropping the new ceramics was worth it for every moment of joy on her face. Of course, a big part of it is that she likes to do what we're doing, but I like to think that another part of it is that it's just fun to drink tea—to discover new tastes, use cute cups, and do it together.

One of my only parenting philosophies is that the best way to make sure that a baby is happy is to be in a good place yourself. You can share the things you love—music, books, foods, and tea—together trying to find songs, foods, and teas that you both like, rather than delineating an option for the child and an option for the adult.

Evening Tea with Children

At some point, Mona was having trouble getting to sleep and staying asleep, and I had my own stressors. I decided to start a chamomile tea evening ritual for the two of us. Shortly after dinner, I would say "It's almost tea-time!" She would get excited, get to choose her cup, and help me set the table. I love chamomile tea for children. Chamomile is so gentle, pretty, and settling. It's calming and good for upset stomachs. Chamomile flowers, both delicate and resilient, are sweet symbols of childhood. I let her participate in the setup by doing things like holding my hand as I pour the tea, cleaning up any spills with a tea towel, and cheering with the cups. When I make tea for my family, I put two ice cubes in the cup for my daughter and pour her tea over it so that hers is ready to drink at the same time as ours.

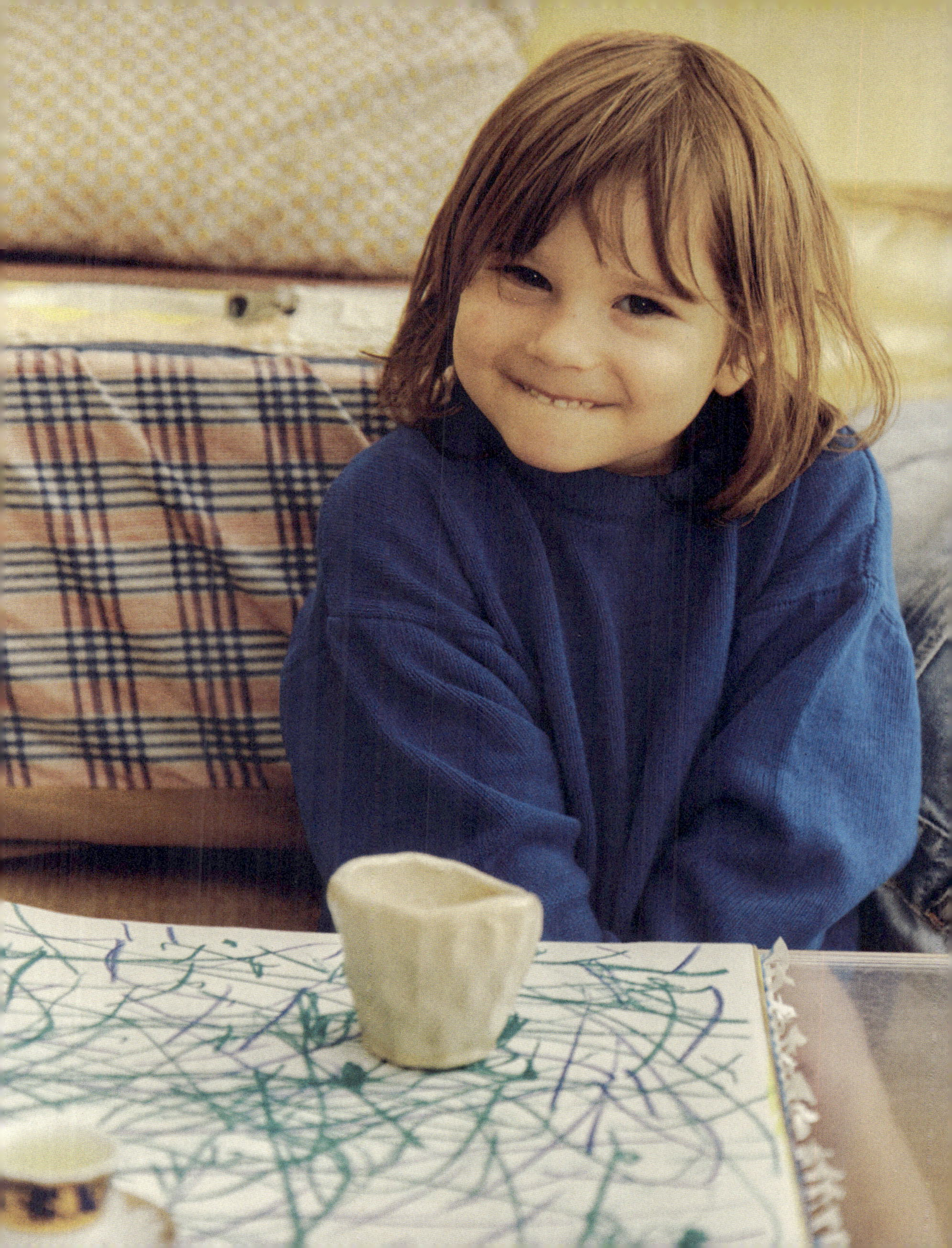

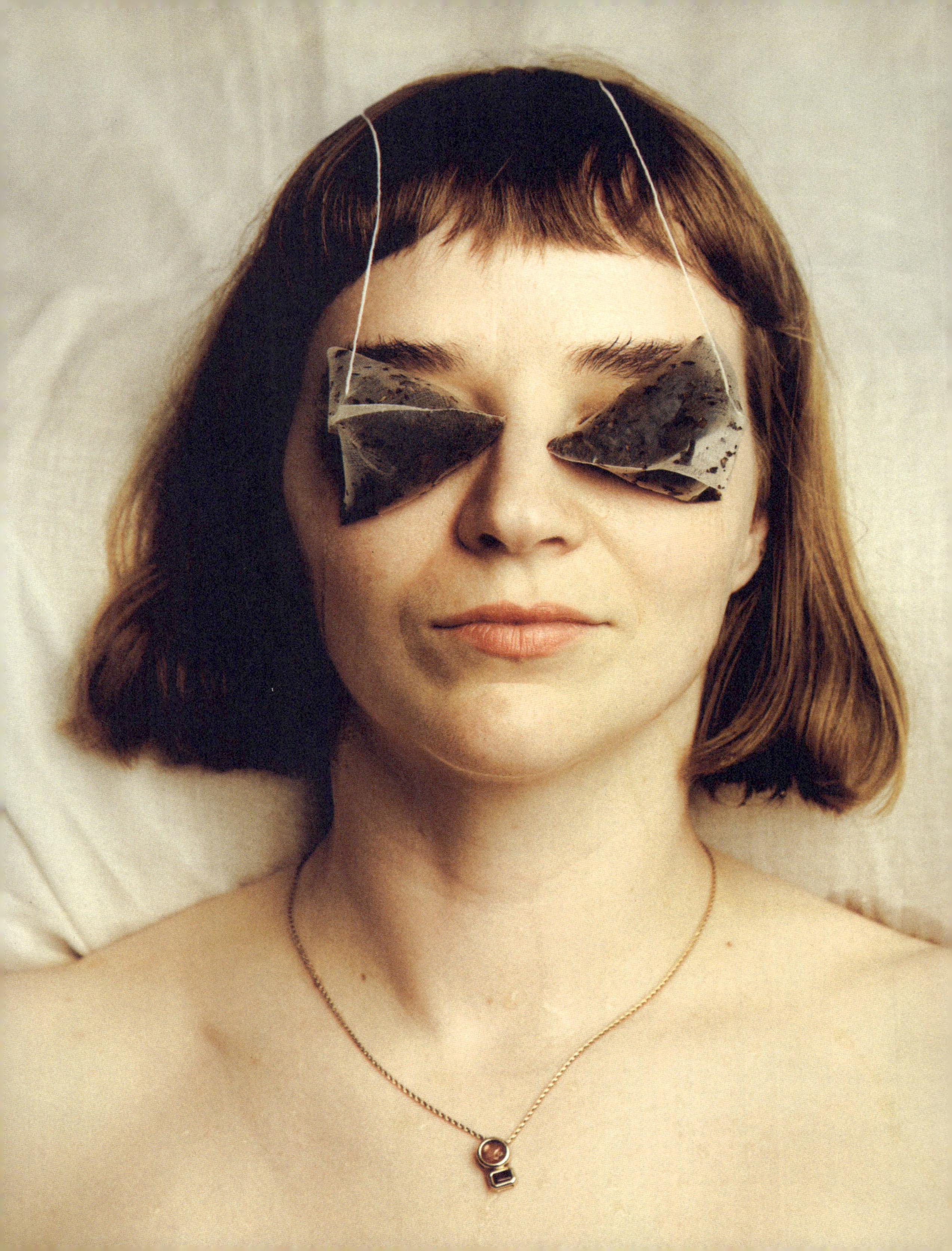

Part 3

Tea and Health

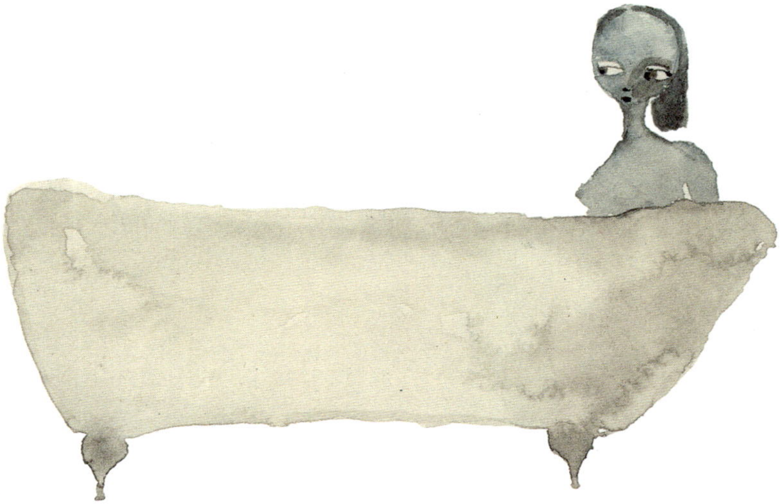

“Who has seen the wind?
Neither I nor you:
But when the leaves hang trembling,
The wind is passing through.

Who has seen the wind?
Neither you nor I:
But when the trees bow down their heads,
The wind is passing by.”
—Christina Rosetti,
“Who Has Seen the Wind” (1872)

– 11 –

Naturopathic Medicine

Tea and naturopathic medicine go hand in hand. While there are specific therapeutic approaches in naturopathy, it is undeniable that the principles surrounding tea culture—slowing down, aligning with nature, and eating whole foods—are also essential naturopathic principles. Aside from healing from a specific illness, naturopathic principles provide structure for a life well-lived. Tea should be enjoyed every day, just for the sake of it. But there are moments where specific teas can be beneficial for you.

A doctorate of naturopathic medicine (ND) is a clinical doctorate encompassing herbal medicine, nutrition, homeopathy, physical medicine, and modern pharmacology and lab testing.

Naturopathic medicine takes a holistic approach, which means looking at all aspects of a person's life when trying to understand why they are unwell. The questions a naturopathic doctor might ask encompass everything from physical, mental, spiritual, and economic issues. There are so many layers to what makes us well or unwell. Holistic practitioners ask themselves if an immediate fix is possible, and, if so, what modality might be least invasive to make that happen. If a quick fix isn't possible, what needs to happen to get to the root of an issue. If it's going to take a long time to address, is there anything that can be done in the interim to make the person's condition more tolerable.

I came to naturopathic medicine in a roundabout way. During my college study abroad program in India, one month of the semester was devoted entirely to an independent study project. I wrote mine on paradigms of Indian medicine, and spent hours shadowing three doctors in the village. As with many Ayurvedic centers, patients stayed for weeks, with prescriptions for daily routines, diets, and herbal treatments. The Ayurvedic garden was the first time I saw herbs grown for medicine. Other than various roses, they were mostly plants I couldn't identify and had never seen before. We spent hours in the garden discussing the various plants and their uses.

After college, I went to medical school in New Jersey, transferring after two years to a naturopathic medical school. After visiting Oregon, I decided to move there and completed medical school in Portland. I lived there for four years. I led herb walks in my downtime. Herbs can be used in developing pharmaceuticals, as supplements, and in tinctures. For me, I 've always liked to keep it simple. I made tea.

Folk Medicine

Folk medicine refers to regional customs for healing, often passed down through oral tradition. Naturopathic medicine has its roots in folk medicine, specifically in Western herbalism. Naturopathic medicine today examines folk medicine through a modern lens, keeping the remedies that work and using them alongside contemporary medical models. Whereas folk medicine is a system of home remedies and apprentice-style medical training, naturopathic medicine integrates that ancient wisdom with modern lab testing, scientific research, and studies evaluating the integrity and accuracy of ancient practices.

The naturopathic medicine that we study in medical schools in the United States teaches mostly German traditions: herbs, hydrotherapy, and homeopathy. Many of these practices, and even the herbs themselves, were similar throughout Europe, and so I turn also to my personal family history, Ashkenazi Judaism, and the folk traditions that have since been written down, studied, and carried on. Folk medicine speaks to the countryside—to self-sufficiency but also community wisdom. With modernization, many scientists shunned folk wisdom, arguing that folk medicine and modern science are mutually exclusive. Now, as researchers begin to allocate funds to study these traditions, we are finding that sometimes tradition precedes science and can be confirmed by it. I believe in ancient wisdom, and in practices that have stood the test of time.

The Elements and Tea

Western herbalism traditionally references four elements: water, fire, air, and earth. There are also paradigms in Eastern medicine for thinking about the elements. Five-Element Acupuncture in Traditional Chinese Medicine, for example, includes the elements fire, water, earth, metal, and wood. Ayurveda includes the three doshas: vata, pitta, and kapha. Vata relates to air, pitta to fire, and kapha to earth. Ayurveda's five elements are vayu (air), jala (water), aakash (space or ether), prithvi (earth), and teja (fire).

It's possible to cultivate an intuitive understanding of ourselves and those around us in relation to the elements. To do so requires learning to observe small details about ourselves and the people around us.

When it comes to working with elements and tea, we think about balance. If you tend to run cold, you might benefit from warming herbs. If you are feeling out of touch with yourself and ungrounded, you might benefit from earth-element herbs. While the five-element system in acupuncture involves seasons and relationships among the elements, for example, wood represents the seasonal cycle of spring and fire represents summer—the symbolism being that wood comes before fire, and feeds fire—the naturopathic perspective, my approach to tea, comes from my specific background in Western herbalism. Below are some considerations with tea and the elements.

WATER: For great tea, you need clean water, whether that be spring or filtered. With delicate Japanese green teas, or subtle wild herbs like rose and juniper, this is especially important.

FIRE: Herbs associated with fire are warming, such as herbs that are in chai, like ginger, cardamom, and clove, and roasted teas like hōjicha.

AIR: This element is associated with floral teas. I would think of delicate flowers like jasmine, chamomile, and lavender for this element. These tend to be soothing and calming.

EARTH: Roots like burdock, licorice, and yellow dock relate to the Earth element. These can make us feel grounded and nourished.

Getting Healthy

There are myriad approaches in natural medicine. If someone is having issues with sleep, for example, approaches could range from massage to herbs, nutritional changes, and pharmacological intervention. A naturopathic doctor spends at least an hour with a patient on the first visit, to understand the full story and symptom picture, and creates a plan that encompasses one or several modalities. Tea is within the herbal and nutritional categories but it can be an adjunctive to other healthy-lifestyle approaches.

As much as marketing efforts will have you think otherwise, tea will not make you lose weight. The only way to lose weight naturally is the old-fashioned way: eating well and exercising. Tea can be a part of that, because it can help regulate stress, which can prevent stress-eating, it can be hydrating, and it can even help with the creation of a tea ritual that can promote regular exercising and mealtimes. Tea is also calorie-free (unless you add milk or sugar), so it can be readily enjoyed during weight loss.

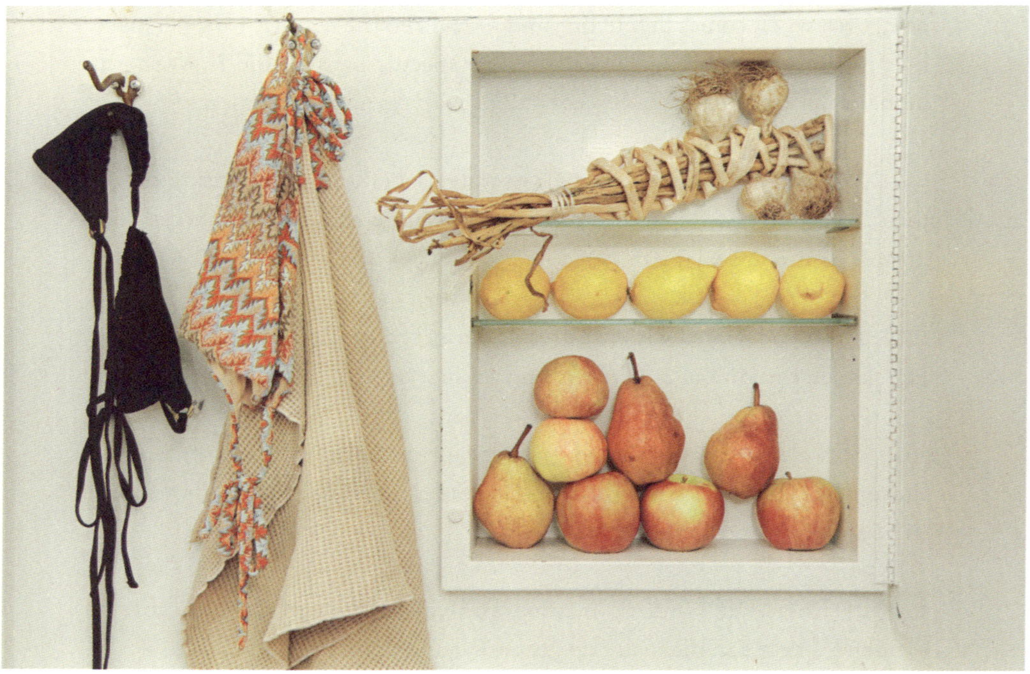

Nutrition

This is an obvious component of health and healing. A whole-foods diet, a seasonal diet full of fresh, organic food with minimal processed food, will invariably be the recommendation from a naturopath. With more specific cases, digestive issues, immune disorders, or even women's health-related complaints, more individualized diets might be suggested. The beauty of tea is that it can be a part of any nutritional routine, whether generally for wellness or more specifically for a particular ailment.

For well-being, the naturopathic approach to nutrition is: Eat simple-ingredient real food, like chicken soup, steamed vegetables, and fresh herbs. Drink tea with real ingredients and whole plants, rather than obscure flavorings and additives.

Botanical Medicine

Botanical medicine, also called herbalism or phytotherapy, refers to the medicinal use of plants. Herbs are used worldwide, across cultures. Medical systems, including pharmacology, naturopathic medicine, Ayurveda, Traditional Chinese Medicine, aromatherapy, and homeopathy all use plants in various ways.

Phytochemistry

This study of the biochemical composition of plants is essential knowledge for developing pharmaceuticals from plants, isolating compounds to make supplements, and helping scientists understand plants' uses and functions. Below are structures that make up the tea plant, *Camellia sinensis*:

CAFFEINE: Several unrelated plant species contain caffeine. Among them, coffee (*coffea* spp.), maté (*Ilex paraguariensis*), cacao (*Theobroma cacao*), and tea (*Camellia sinensis*). Caffeine is a diuretic, and it has a stimulating effect on the respiratory, cardiovascular, and nervous system. It's a component of some aspirin and acetaminophen pills to aid in pain relief.

THEOBROMINE: A central nervous system and circulatory stimulant, also found in the cocoa plant.

THEOPHYLLINE: Although it's found naturally (in small quantities) in tea, because it structurally resembles caffeine it is often synthesized by chemists from the caffeine molecule for use in medicine. Theophylline, in much higher quantities than those found in the tea plant, and together with other drugs, is available by prescription as a bronchodilator, used to treat symptoms of asthma, emphysema, and chronic bronchitis. It is a quick-acting diuretic and cardiac stimulant.

TANNINS: The name "tannin" comes from the ability of tannic compounds to convert animal hide to leather. Tannins are found in all parts of plants, from roots to stems and leaves. Tannins have medicinal uses ranging from protecting inflamed mucous membranes to reducing inflammation during infections.

CATECHINS: These are antioxidants. The ones found in green tea include epigallocatechin (EGC) and epigallocatechin-3-gallate (EGCG). Studies on the use of green tea in cancer prevention focus on the catechins EGC and EGCG specifically. Because green tea is less processed than black, oolong, or pu'erh, it has the highest amount of these anti-inflammatory catechins.

Hydrotherapy

Naturopathic hydrotherapy refers to the use of water to facilitate healthy blood circulation and healing. This can be through baths, mineral springs, compresses, poultices, castor oil packs, and alternating hot and cold.

Cultural Applications

Banyas, onsens, Turkish baths, natural hot springs—sauna culture prevails around the world for the immediacy of its feel-good effects, for the long-term health benefits, and for the sensory experience. Saunas are restorative, grounding, and sometimes community building. Almost universally, tea accompanies sauna culture. While saunas warm from the outside, tea warms internally.

I spent a winter living in Saratoga, Wyoming, where the natural hot spring in the middle of town is open to the public. The history of the springs involved three local Indigenous tribes, the Cheyenne, Ute, and Arapaho, who recognized the healing properties of the hot springs and called it "the place of magic water." It was neutral ground, a place of peace and conflict resolution.

Growing up in an Eastern European household, after skiing we would go in the hot tub, then jump in the snow, and return to the hot tub, and so on. This example of cold plunging shows how these principles can be applied in a fun, culturally relevant way.

Hydrotherapy at Home

At home, there are several ways to use hydrotherapy and to complement the treatment with tea. Many forms of hydrotherapy raise core body temperature. Tea can support this process by warming the body from the inside. Hydrotherapy treatments themselves can often be stimulating with the sudden changes in temperature. After the treatment, tea is beneficial in helping to wind down and conclude on a relaxing note.

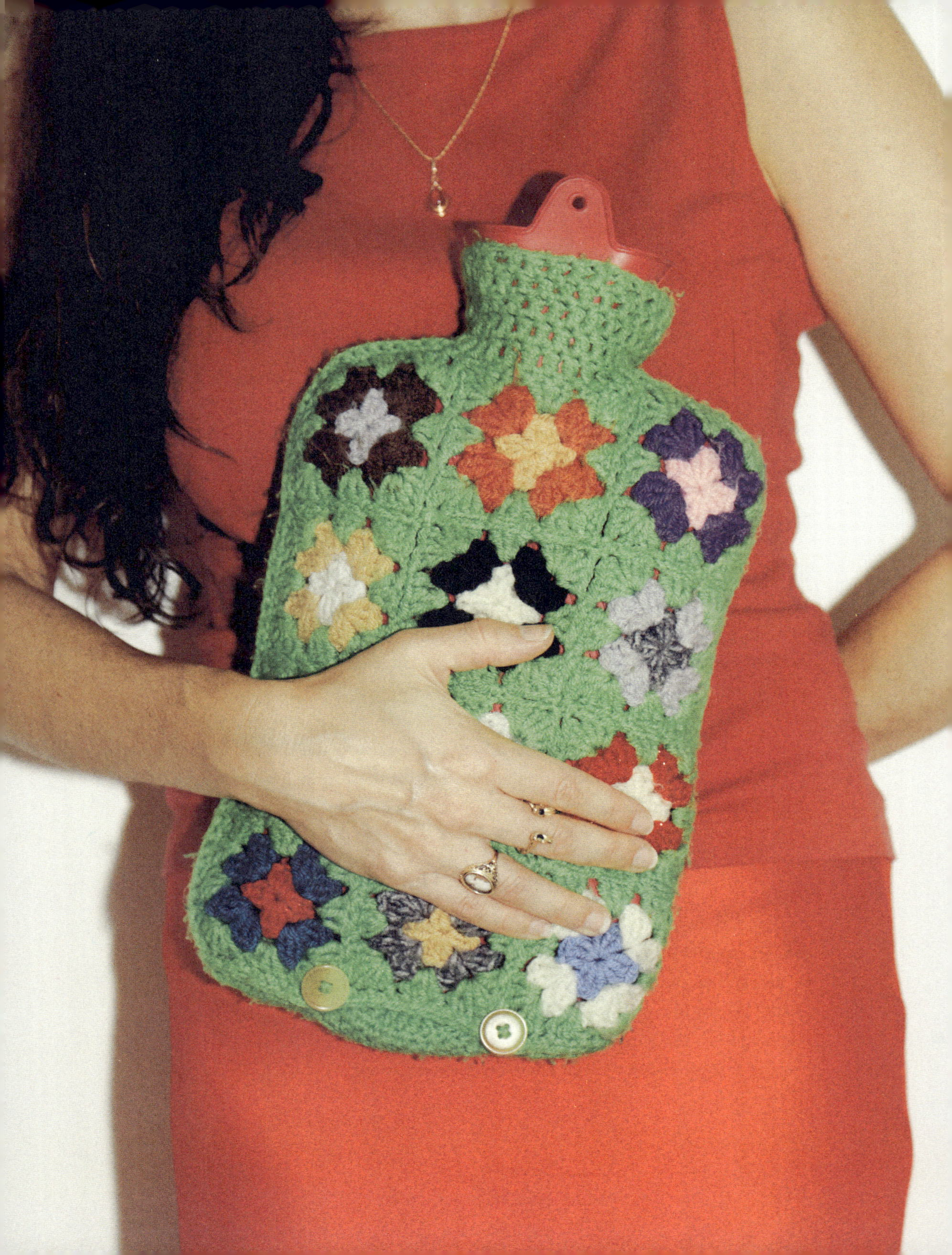

HOT WATER BOTTLE: A simple rubber bottle, ideally covered with wool or some other heavy fabric, can help soothe menstrual complaints like cramps, but also digestive upset or just feeling cold in the winter.

HOT FOOT BATH: Mostly used for headaches, a hot foot bath is best accompanied by a cold towel or icepack on the forehead or back of the neck. The idea is to stimulate circulation. Heat causes blood vessels to open up (in this case in the lower extremities) and the ice causes blood vessels to constrict (in this case in the head and neck), decreasing headache pain and inflammation.

STEAM INHALATION: Ideal for opening up the upper airways, this feels so soothing for a cold or cough. The same idea is used in opening up the pores for beauty rituals. Steam inhalation involves pouring hot water into a bowl, and then putting your face over the bowl (not touching the water, and keeping your eyes closed), with a towel overhead to create steam. This can be completed with essential oils, tea, or fresh herbs in the water (see How to Make an Herbal Steam, page 213).

COLD PLUNGE: Best after a sauna or soak in a hot tub, the point of a cold plunge is to stimulate circulation. A way to apply this principle at home is to end a shower with cold water. In naturopathic hydrotherapy, sometimes alternating hot and cold packs are applied to the chest or other parts of the body. With that, the general rule is to always end with cold.

WARMING SOCKS: A favorite naturopathic technique for overcoming respiratory infections, you'll need two pairs of socks: cotton and wool. The cotton socks should be ice cold (which can be achieved by soaking them in ice water). First, take a shower or bath. Immediately after drying off, put on the ice-cold cotton socks (these should not be dripping wet), covered by a pair of dry wool socks and get into bed under the covers. You can fall asleep like this or leave them on for at least 20 minutes. This stimulates circulation and creates a robust immune response for faster healing.

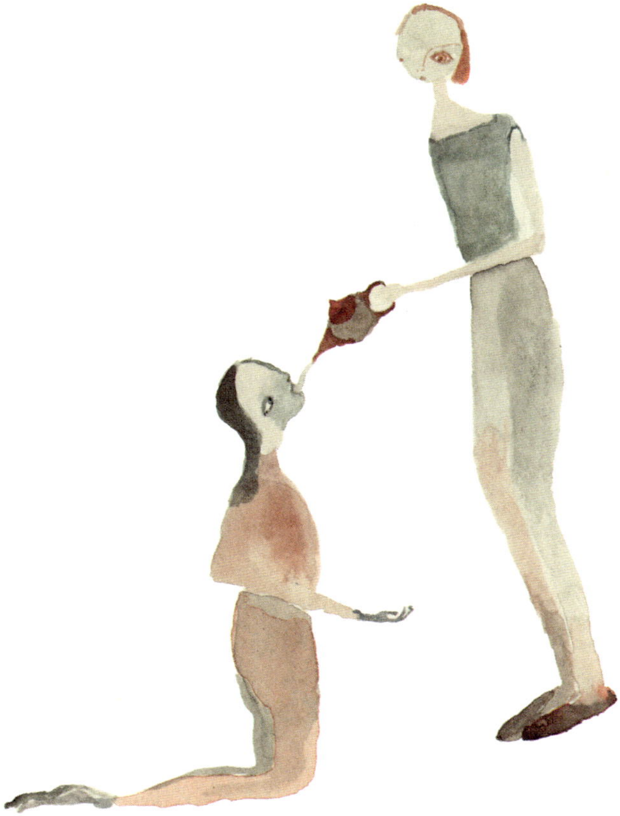

"I am sorry to say that Peter was not very well during the evening. His mother put him to bed, and made some chamomile tea; and she gave a dose of it to Peter! 'One table-spoonful to be taken at bed-time.' But Flopsy, Mopsy, and Cotton-tail had bread and milk and blackberries for supper."

—Beatrix Potter, *Peter Rabbit* (1901)

– 12 –

Healing Teas

From the onset, teas and herbs have been valued for their medicinal benefits. For specific conditions, it's always best to consult with a licensed provider, like a naturopath or acupuncturist, to create a specific herbal treatment plan. At the same time, with some understanding about how to approach healing teas, you can learn to use teas to bring the restorative elements of the natural world into your daily life. Growing herbs, building a pantry, and blending teas are foundational to then understanding the different properties that herbs can have in supporting the health of body systems. Unlike drugs or supplements that isolate specific biochemical compounds, teas have hundreds of herbal constituents, making them useful for gently supporting your whole system to achieve balance.

When it comes to tea, *Camellia sinensis* leaves are processed and harvested quite intentionally. Tea leaves are picked in autumn for hōjicha, grown under the shade for matcha, and left out to oxidize for black tea. Sometimes after this, tea leaves are fermented, in the case of pu'erh, or smoked in pine, in the case of lapsang souchong. In tea-growing parts of the world, families may have small tea gardens beside their homes. In other parts of the world, herbal gardens—whether outdoors, in a community garden, or even on a windowsill—are possible. One way of harnessing the healing power of tea and herbs is through gardening, which helps us understand and visualize how they grow. Especially for people who live in cities, reconnecting with the natural world can be key to healing. Understanding that natural materials, like teas, come from nature is a great place to begin. An alternative way to be active in the processing is to dry your own herbs. Ideally, you get a bouquet of herbs at the farmers market and then hang them upside down to dry in your kitchen. You can cut the dried herbs for use at home.

Finding Herbs and Flowers at Farmers Markets

Going to a farmers market is a way to contextualize the place you live within the greater geography of the region. In New York City in mid-May, exciting fresh herbs and flowers come to the farmers market. It's a profound shift from the potatoes and beets of winter. I love to buy flowers then and bring them home to make bouquets; I also make teas from the flowers that can be used for this purpose. In mid-May, just toward the end of ramp season—ramps are probably the most popular foraged food in New York, and as such have suffered from overharvesting—comes another favorite foraged tea component, spruce tips. Spruce trees grow fresh, light-green sprouts at their "tips" every spring, and foragers cut them for use in cooking, beer brewing, and for making tea. Regarding spruce tips and some of the other market delights that can be used for tea, I love them most for their beautiful shapes or colors, more than for flavoring the tea itself. I use things like spruce tips in a layering way: I might make a cup of black tea with one spruce tip bud, just to experience the smell and the color, more than to affect the flavor of the tea. This layering is akin to painting with different shades of the same color.

Around the same time, chamomile flowers come, so delightful with their oversized yellow centers and delicate white petals. A bunch bought from the market might only make one to three cups of tea, but those cups of tea are so worth it, and in between or before they become cups of tea, they serve as table flowers for adornment. Stinging nettle also comes to the market in the spring—a useful herb that grows abundantly as a weed. I'm sure that most of the farms that come to market are foraging their nettle versus growing it for harvest, though herb farms do cultivate nettle. Nettle has long been used to aid with seasonal allergies and so it grows at the perfect time. Other herbs that I love to get at the market for fresh tea include mint, with its dozens of varieties, as well as holy basil, lemon balm, and shiso. Shiso tea, in particular, retains its complex herbal flavor when prepared with the fresh herb, especially when cold-brewed.

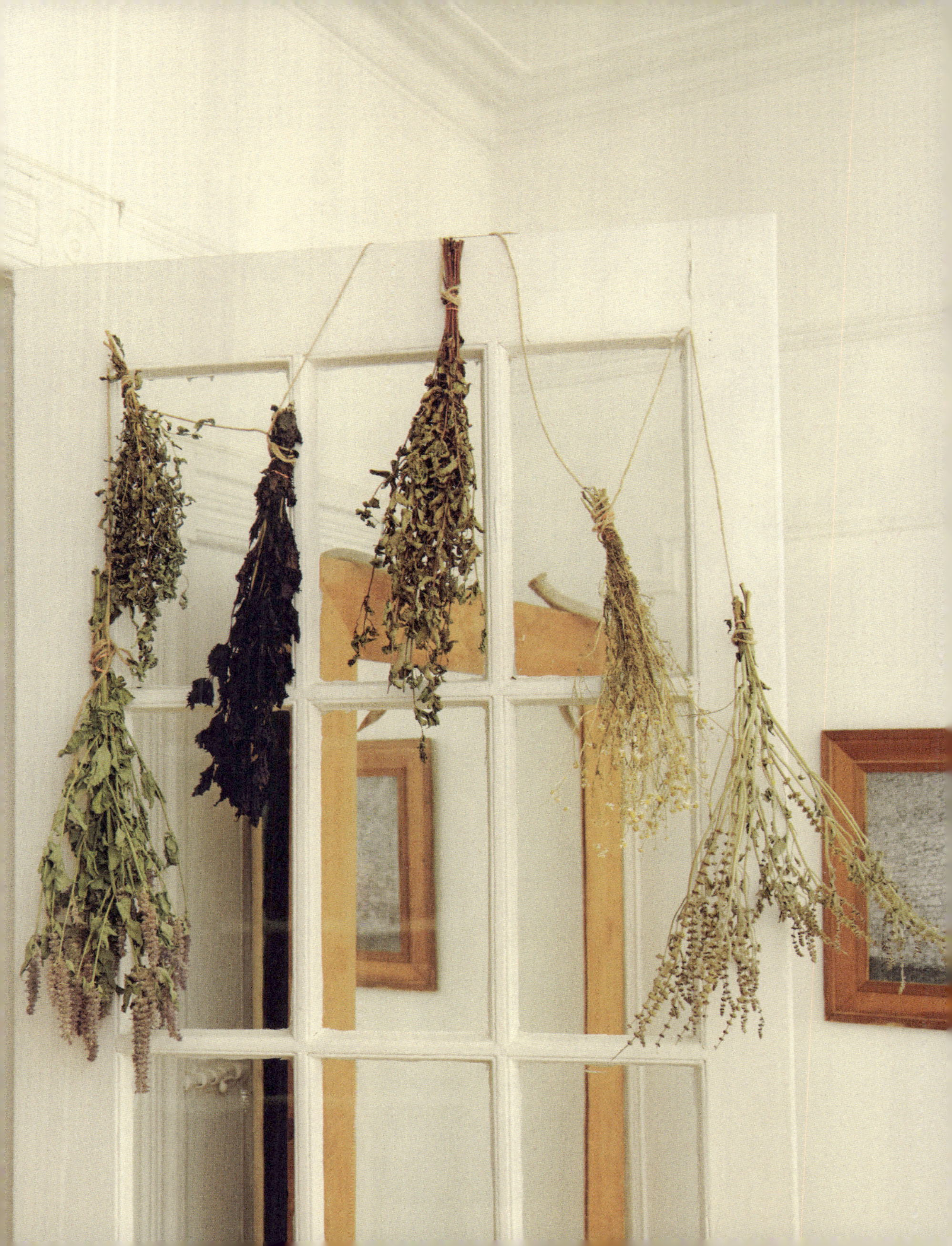

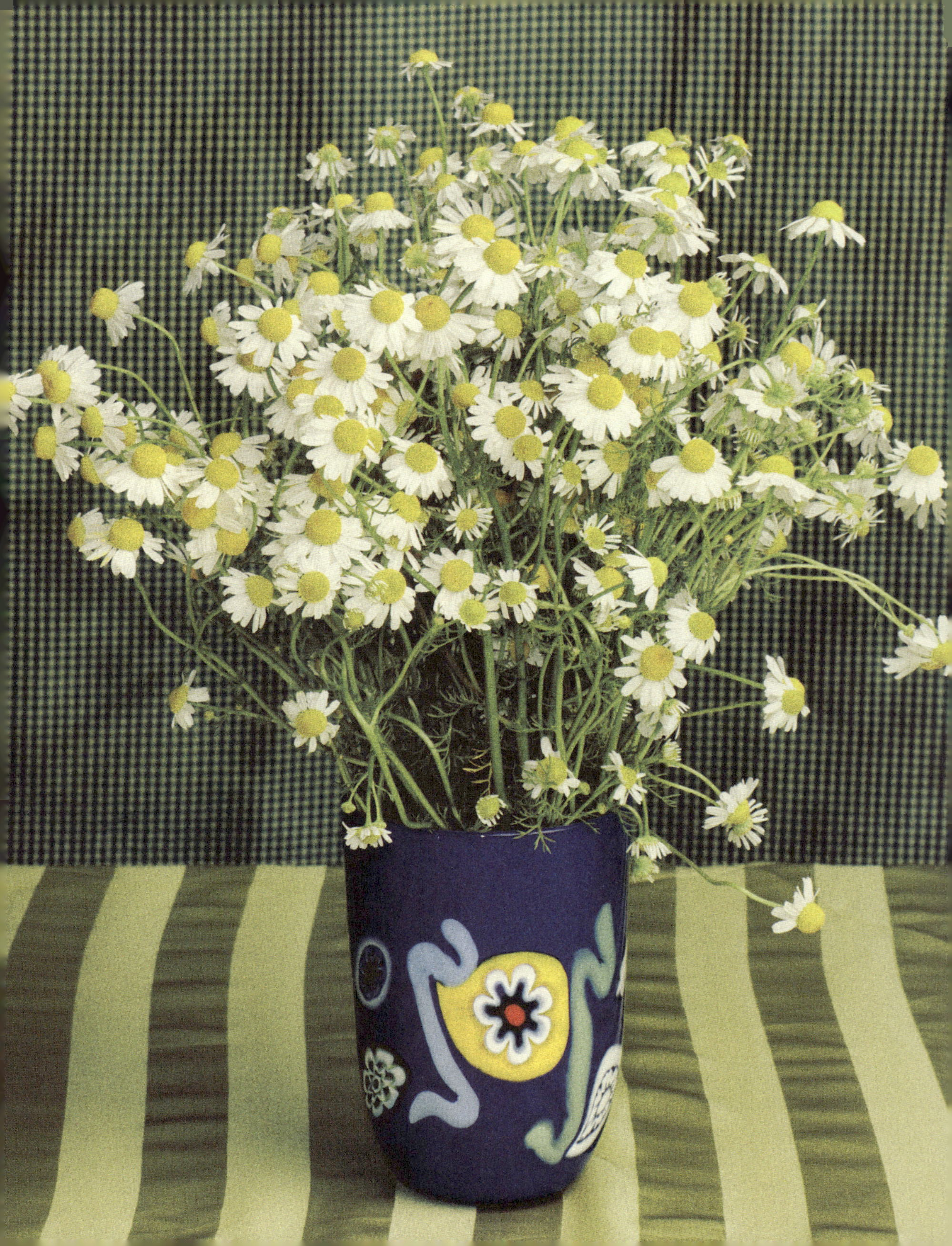

How to Find Your Comfort Herbs

Tea has been boiled, whisked, and steeped for centuries. Some consider tea making an art form, capable of becoming a masterpiece or just another piece of bad art. Others are less precious about it, and still others dedicate their lives to tea accoutrements: many potters, writers, and artists have considered tea central to their work. Generations of farmers have dedicated their lives to the simple plant, and there have been periods of time when certain teas have been more expensive per ounce than solid gold.

Anyone can make a healing cup of tea, which can be therapeutic for many reasons. It can warm you up when you have a cold, it can be prepared in a cup that a loved one gave you, providing a moment to remember the person, it can be hydrating. If you have a basic understanding of even a handful of herbs, you can select teas that might be beneficial for you at a specific moment of the day, like before bed or first thing in the morning, or a moment in time, like a stressful period at work or when overcoming an illness. It isn't necessary to become an herbalist or to study dozens of plants to do this. Finding even a few herbs that work for you and your body is sufficient.

The best way to explore this is to make a cup of tea with a single herb and notice how you feel. Do you like how it smells, tastes, or even looks? What does it remind you of? If you identify one or two plants that make you feel calm, grounded, or at ease, that is useful information. Because then, even if you're wanting to make a tea to help with something specific, such as overcoming a cold, you can always include one of your comfort herbs to make a blend. In this way, you can personalize your tea blends and make them work for you.

In the same way that you build a pantry in your kitchen, where you might always have olive oil, salt, oats, and so on, you can thus build a base of teas. This might mean that you always have one black, one green, and one herbal tea at home. Or, it might mean that you always have your two comfort teas in the cabinet. That way, even if you have special or extra teas, from travels or something that you want to try, you'll always have your tried-and-true favorite teas to blend with, or to have on their own when you need.

Choosing Herbs for Tea

The following are the main teas that I like to drink, blend, and use, here organized based on feeling. While everybody reacts to plants differently, there are certain ubiquitous effects that certain plants have on people. Imagine lying on the ground in a lavender farm looking up at the sky listening to honeybees, inhaling the smell, catching glimpses of the purple flowers dancing in the wind; you wouldn't soon forget how that experience made you feel. The smell and taste of lavender gets us to that place, even if subconsciously.

The list of herbs brewed as teas across cultures and traditions is vast. There are important ones that I've left out—jasmine, cinnamon, and passionflower, to name a few—but this selection is based on the plants that I most frequently turn to, both for my tea company and for use at home. Technically, only *Camellias*, in the family Theaceae, are truly tea, and all the other herbs listed below are tisanes, but it's common practice today to call them herbal teas.

The teas and herbs in this chapter are categorized into six feelings—grounding, warming, cooling, calming, romantic, and resilient.

-one-

Grounding

Rooted in place, confident with the steps we're taking, feeling down to earth and present in our bodies: these are feelings of groundedness. This can be so hard to achieve when we're burdened with responsibilities, with the desire to move forward, with the incentive to rush to catch up to an envisioned future. Buddhist monks started drinking tea because it helped them meditate. What is meditation if not being present? For that reason, I categorized tea, true tea, in this section, alongside a root (literally grounded in the soil), and several evergreen trees. One of the most frequent comments that I get when I mention trees in my tea blends is, "I didn't know you could make tea from that." Evergreen forests are powerful places. You are enveloped by the sight, smell, color, and movement of living beings that can live for hundreds to thousands of years. It's disarming and brings you down to earth.

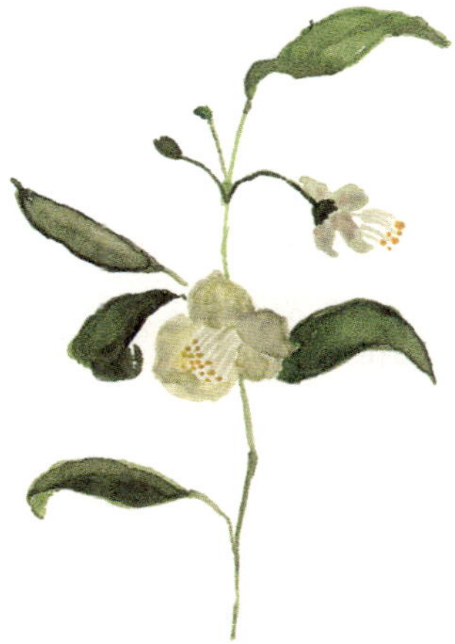

TEA

Camellia sinensis

"When we consider how small after all the cup of human enjoyment is, how soon overflowed with tears . . . Why not consecrate ourselves to the queen of the Camellias, and revel in the warm stream of sympathy that flows from her altar?"
—Kakuzō Okakura, *The Book of Tea* (1906)

Tea is an evergreen shrub. From the same *Camellia sinensis*, farmers produce black, green, hōjicha, matcha, oolong, pu'erh, and white teas. The difference is how these teas are processed. *Camellia sinensis* contains caffeine, and so is a stimulant, but the caffeine content is determined by oxidation, with black teas having the highest caffeine content and white teas having the least.

Black Tea

Black tea undergoes the longest process of oxidation (exposure to air before being heated to stop the process). Oxidation can involve bruising, rolling, or tumbling the leaves after picking them. Black tea is oxidized for up to twelve hours to achieve 80 to 100 percent oxidation.

Green

Green tea is the most minimally oxidized as the teas are heated almost immediately after picking. The Chinese and Japanese style of processing green tea differs in that the heating process in the Chinese style involves roasting, whereas the Japanese steam the tea leaves—and these different styles impact the flavor profile. Roasted tea creates more nutty, mellow notes, whereas steaming creates vegetal, grassy notes. Outside of Japan, most other tea-growing regions, like India and Kenya, adopted the Chinese style. Because I source green teas mostly from Japan for Masha Tea, *Nihoncha*, or Japanese tea, is the style that I am more familiar with.

Green tea is high in antioxidants. Antioxidants help in preventing many chronic diseases and also in keeping skin healthy. Pharmacists and beauty brands, in particular, have included green tea in skincare formulations for these properties.

Oolong

This tea falls somewhere between black and green tea in terms of oxidation. After oxidation, oolong tea is rolled and roasted. Rolling the tea gives it its signature oblong shape and releases more flavor. Oolongs are complex and can vary greatly in color and flavor based on the production style.

Pu'erh

Pu'erh is a hand-processed tea that is stored in disc shapes called bricks or cakes, packed in rice paper, and aged anywhere from months to years in caves. Microorganisms ferment this tea and there are two main styles—Sheng and Shu. Sheng is made with raw green tea leaves and Shu is made from black tea.

White

White tea contains tea leaves that are withered and dried without the application of heat. The flavor can be subtle, which makes sense given that it is harvested by hand as new buds of emerging leaves. Because it is minimally processed, white tea contains the highest antioxidant content of all teas, even more than green.

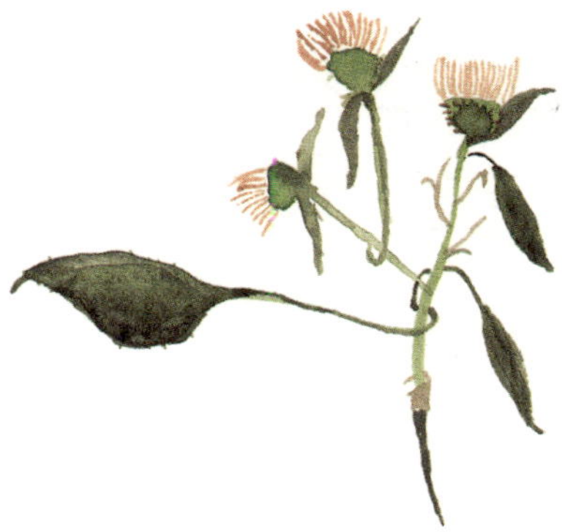

BURDOCK

Arctium lappa

To make tea from burdock, the burdock root, also called *gobo,* is cut, sifted, and dried and imparts a grounded, earthy flavor. You can tell that you're drinking a root versus a leaf from the heavy, thick texture of the tea. Burdock has a robust flavor profile on its own, both when served hot or iced. I think of this plant as generally healthy and nourishing, supporting liver detoxification pathways and thereby digestion. When blending burdock, consider other roots or rhizomes, like licorice, turmeric, or ginger, or herbs with a similarly earthy flavor, like echinacea or nettle. Burdock is used worldwide across herbal traditions.

The alterative category of herbs, of which burdock is a part, supports detoxification. In naturopathic medicine, we refer to the organs of elimination as the *emunctories*—these include the skin, digestive tract, urinary tract, and lungs. With skin issues like acne, eczema, and psoriasis, the naturopathic approach is to support all of the emunctory organs, starting with the digestive tract and liver. Alterative herbs help do that. Because a result of this support is healthy digestion, clearing skin often follows. Along with alteratives, additional naturopathic liver support can include simple at-home practices like castor oil packs, hot water bottles, and exercise followed by the sauna.

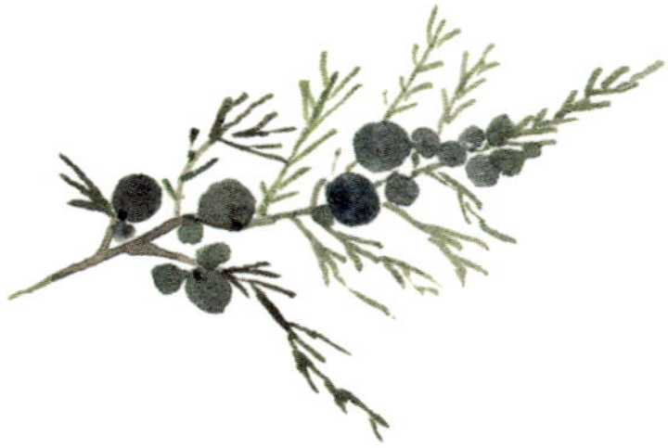

JUNIPER

Juniperus communis

For tea, I use both the berries and the stems, typically cut at an inch or two from the tip. Like cedar, opposite, juniper is in the *Cupresseceae* (cypress) family and extracts better in alcohol than water, so it is more of an aesthetic choice in tea blends, due to both its smell and the beauty of its branches, versus a flavor-forward one. Because juniper is used subtly, it blends well with other aromatic, evocative herbs like tulsi and mint, which have strong smells, too, but also strong flavors that can carry the blend. *Medicinal note:* Juniper is used for urinary-tract complaints.

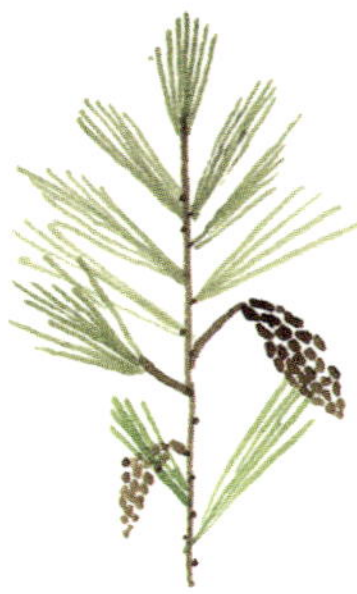

PINE

Pinus

When I think of pine, I remember the smell of my dad's chessboard, which is made of pinewood and still somehow smells decades after he first got it. Think of your memories with plants, and their smells, and consider if there is a way to incorporate them into teas for their grounding effects. Consider the shape of pine needles and how they feel. These properties translate to the cup of tea. Pine needle tea smells like the forest and tastes subtle. Pine can be blended with green or white tea to enhance fragrance. I have blended pine with green tea and cherry blossoms to invoke springtime.

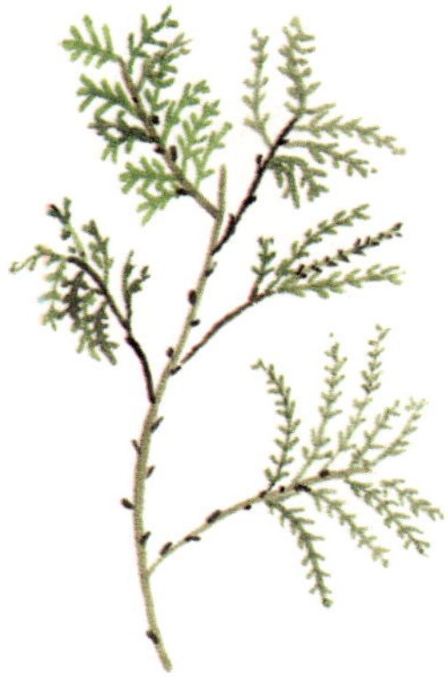

CEDAR

Thuja plicata

Western red cedar, an evergreen member of the cypress family, is native to the American Pacific Northwest. The active constituents are soluble in alcohol, not water, so for a tea, it primarily contributes smell and texture. For many of the high-essential-oil plants, like cedar, the hot water on them releases the smells, but it doesn't release the flavor. I find this an interesting way to layer a tea. I blend cedar with rose and anise hyssop for the Masha Love Tea. Dried, you might notice the smell of roses. Upon brewing, when you bring it up to your nose, the first thing you notice is the smell of the cedar. While drinking, the main flavor is anise hyssop, with a hint of rose, but what you're smelling when drinking is that deep forest cedar. *Medicinal note:* Cedar is sometimes used for its antifungal properties, though that is more typically delivered in essential oil or topical form.

-two-

Warming

Warming teas get your blood moving and, quite literally, make you feel warm. Many of these are also spices or cooking herbs. Constitutionally, if you are somebody who runs cold, this category of herbs would be beneficial for you. Most familiarly, when blended together, either all or in combination, these aromatic herbs can make a lovely chai.

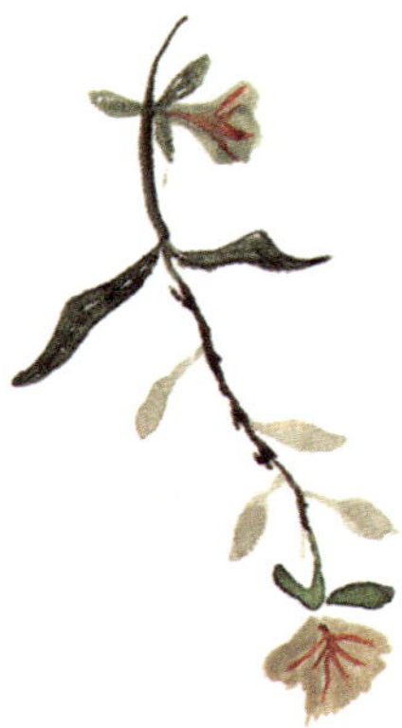

CARDAMOM

Elettaria cardamomum

The smell of cardamom evokes comfort and warmth for me, like cozy, thick blankets in winter. In the same plant family as ginger (Zingerabacea), opposite—a plant family refers to shared characteristics and presumed evolutionary similarities—cardamom is similarly aromatic and spicy. Like ginger, cardamom grows from rhizomes, but while it's the rhizomes themselves that are used in ginger tea, cardamom pods are harvested after about three years of plant growth. After drying and turning brown in the sun, the pods are ready to use. When making tea with cardamom, it's best to crush the pods before steeping them to get the most flavor. You can do this by grinding the cardamom seeds in a grinder or mortar and pestle right before you're going to make the tea. Like the other aromatic herbs, cardamom can be helpful to settle an upset stomach.

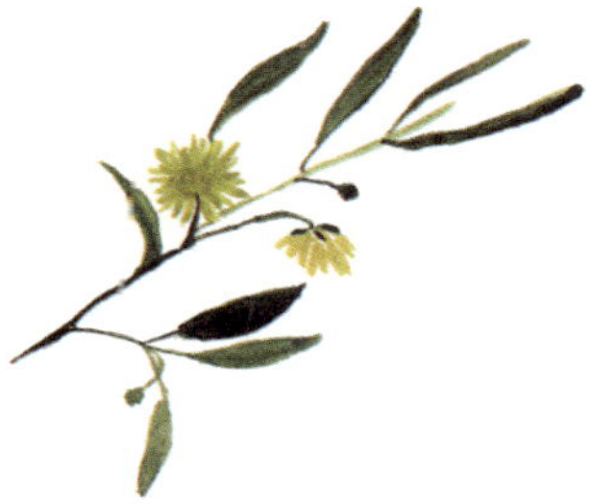

STAR ANISE

Illicium verum

I add star anise to chai blends for its shape, usually an eight-sided star. The robust spice adds a sweet pungency to blends. Star anise is actually a fruit tree indigenous to southern China and Vietnam. The seed pods from the fruit are used medicinally to aid in coughs and also as a digestive support. It makes a delicious and pretty addition to teas. When serving tea that tends toward warm or spicy, it can be fun to put one star anise in the cup for each person so it floats on top for visual effect. It can either be removed before drinking or left in the cup while drinking. Consider pairing with holy basil, black tea, vanilla, clove, and the herbs in this warming section. For a traditional chai, star anise may be ground to release the full extent of its flavor.

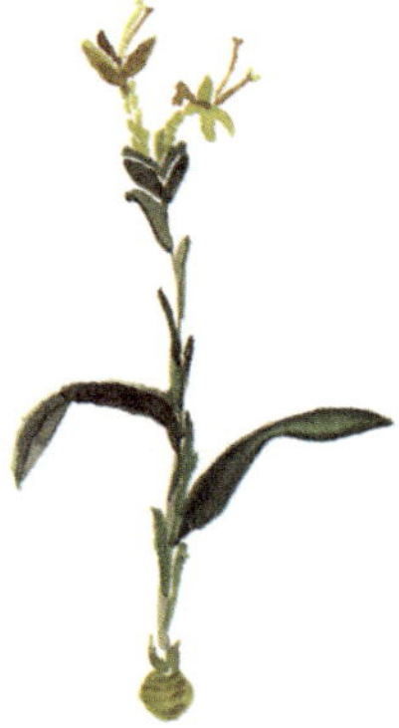

GINGER

Zingiber officinale

Gingerroot, with its distinctive spice and aroma, can be prepared so many ways from a culinary perspective, and for our purposes, brewed to make a deep and lovely tea, prepared with either fresh or dried root. The dried root can be cut up or powdered. *Zingiber officinale* is indigenous to Southeast

Asia, though I have seen it grown under controlled conditions in upstate New York. Though commonly called gingerroot, the part of the plant used is not the root but the rhizome. Ginger is a great entry into home remedies and has a variety of uses. Most simply, ginger can be used as a treatment for upset stomach or nausea, including nausea caused by carsickness. It also has great anti-inflammatory properties. I would prescribe high-dose ginger capsules for my naturopathic patients who suffered from painful periods.

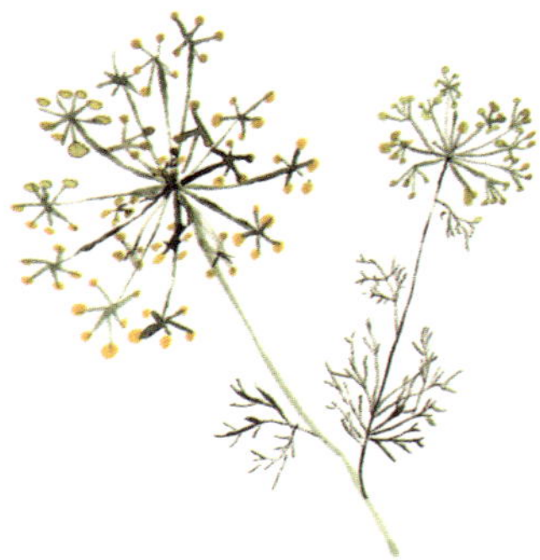

FENNEL

Foeniculum vulgare

Fennel is in the Apiacaea, or parsley, family and grows tall and beautiful in an umbel shape, which kind of looks like an umbrella. The seeds, which have an anise-like flavor, are the part of the plant used for tea. To make fennel tea, pour water over the seeds and consider blending with other herbs that support digestion. I make a tea called Après, a blend of fennel, mint, and licorice, intended for "après" (after) meals to help support digestion. I rarely have fennel tea on its own but rather add fennel for the smell, flavor, and even the sound the dried fennel seeds make when bumping up against one another when stirred with a spoon or poured into a jar. They have a hefty weight to them, too, which makes them enjoyable to handle. I add them to chai blends, but also to anise hyssop and licorice blends. Along with that licorice-like flavor, fennel has a sweetness to it and it can make an ideal after-dinner tea or tea to serve with dessert. Fennel is a carminative herb, meaning it is a digestive aid to prevent bloating or discomfort after a large meal.

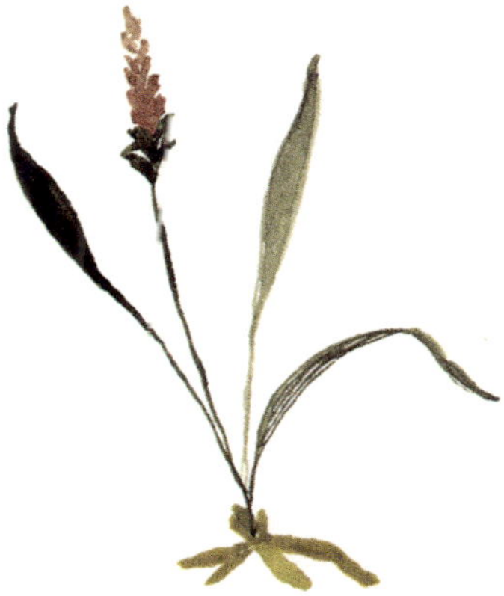

TURMERIC

Curcuma longa

It's impossible to think of turmeric without first considering its bright marigold-yellow color. Most often found powdered in spice cabinets, or in majestic mountain-shaped piles in outdoor markets in India, turmeric root, cut up and dried, makes a subtly sweet and spicy addition to tea blends. The rhizome is used for tea. Curcumin, one of the major constituents of turmeric, is extracted and used for its anti-inflammatory properties. I find the flavor mildly spicy and I often pair it with black pepper when cooking, using it in smoothies, and when making tea blends. For tea, use it for its vibrant color, balancing flavor, and warm earthiness. Turmeric pairs easily with any other spicy flavor, and also with black tea and vanilla, but after tasting a blend with elderflower, I suggest that you consider pairing it with other earthy and even floral partners.

-three-

Cooling

Aside from making delicious iced teas, these plants tend to have a cooling effect on the body, even when served warm. People who tend to run hot temperature-wise, those who relate to the term "coming in hot," may find a sense of balance from these teas. When I start drinking licorice, for example, I will often have several pots of this tea throughout the day because it makes me feel alert, energized, and hydrated.

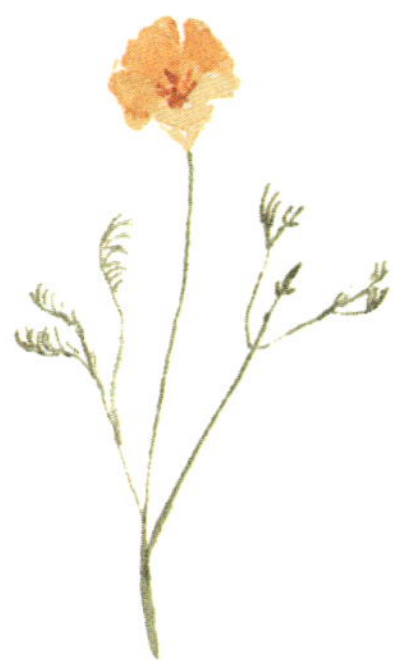

CALIFORNIA POPPY

Eschscholzia californica

California poppy is in the Papaveraceae family, the same powerful family as opium and other opiates. Think of California poppy as the gentle, harmless, calming, and nonaddictive cousin. Bright orange and native to California, consider it a plant for cooling down in the overwhelm of hot summer. Because it is bitter to taste, I actually like to include it more for the sexy name and the evocative image of the flowers growing on a mountainside than for the flavor profile. I still include a small amount in blends with other colorful plants like orange or citrus peel, or alongside other calming plants like lavender and mugwort for an evening tea. I blend California poppy with other herbs to mask most of the bitterness. On the other hand, bitter teas make excellent digestive aids, ideally consumed before meals to stimulate the formation of digestive enzymes and thus ease the digestive process.

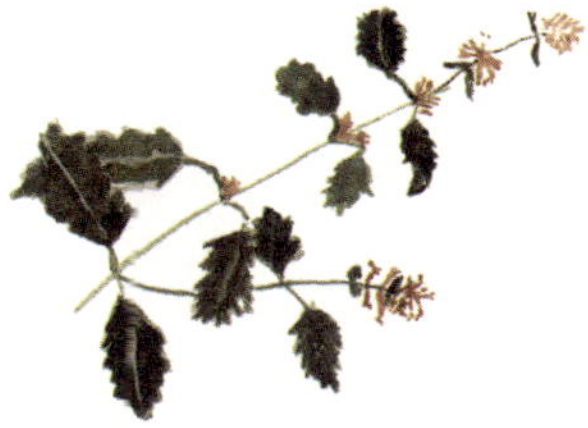

MINT

Mentha spp.

Mint tea is a classic and is the most recognized herbal flavor. The mint family includes peppermint (*Mentha piperita*) and spearmint (*Mentha spicata*), but more unusual mints exist as well: chocolate mint (*Mentha piperita f. citrata*), so named for its dark leaves; water mint (*Mentha aquatica*); and apple mint (*Mentha suaveolens*), to name a few. The leaves are used for tea. Mint tea, a crowd-pleaser, is an easy herbal staple to have in the pantry because people are already familiar with it. While mint is often used for digestive upsets, it should be avoided by those suffering from reflux, as it can exacerbate the condition.

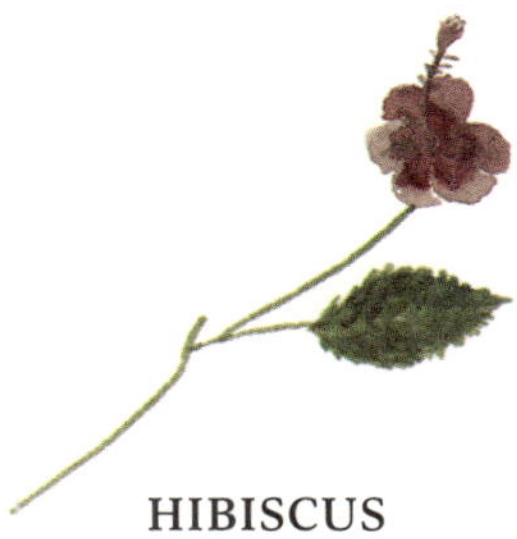

HIBISCUS

Hibiscus rosa-sinensis

The bright red color of hibiscus tea and its tart freshness make it a favorite iced tea across cultures. For tea, we use whole, dried hibiscus flowers. Hot, the color is an even darker red. Every summer my husband keeps a gallon of hibiscus cold brew in the fridge—it's hydrating, flavorful, and matches the brightness of summertime. Because of the strong flavor, hibiscus can overpower blends, but ginger or other equally strong flavors make a super flavorful tea. *Medicinal notes:* Hibiscus supports circulation and the cardiovascular system. For cardiovascular support, it's also important to address nutrition, exercise, and other lifestyle considerations.

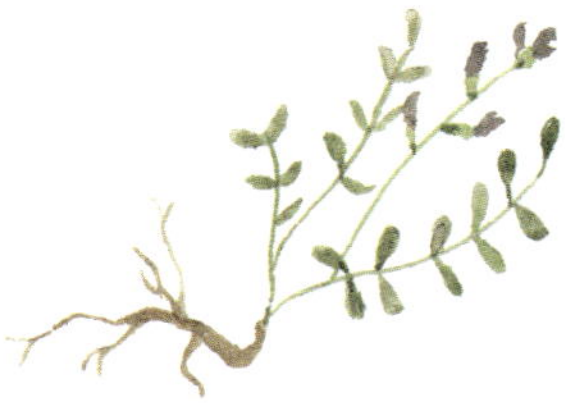

LICORICE

Glycyrrhiza glabra

Licorice-root tea surprises people. Many don't realize the natural sweetness, the richness, and the tongue-coating nature of this root. Demulcent herbs like licorice have a thick texture, a property that you can feel in your throat and back of your mouth when drinking them. Because of this property, it is often used in throat-coat teas, also called singers' teas. In high doses it also has a hormonal effect and is considered for women's health conditions. The root is typically cut and dried when made for tea. The flavor is quite strong and is powerful on its own, so it doesn't really need to be blended to be enjoyed. But if you want to moderate the flavor a bit, you can blend licorice with an earthy burdock or with mint for balance.

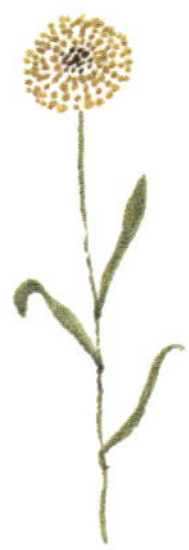

CALENDULA

Calendula officinalis

Gardeners plant calendula, also known as marigold, as an ornamental plant. Tastewise, it's slightly astringent and a touch bitter, despite the pretty blossom. I add calendula flowers to tea for their beauty: the many petals hold on to the plants around them when water is poured over them, bringing a joy and life to the teas that they accompany. I blend calendula with chamomile and lemon balm for a tea I make called Calm, but also with earthier burdock and echinacea for my Earth tea. I also include calendula in bath blends (see page 210).

-four-

Calming

Feeling calm, or the desire to feel calm, to slow down, to step away from the grind of daily life, is a reason people turn to tea culture. Outside of feeling more embodied and comfortable, having a regulated nervous system makes us healthier in every way. While drinking any type of tea, or having any type of meditative experience, can bring calm, I turn specifically to the herbs below to drive that feeling.

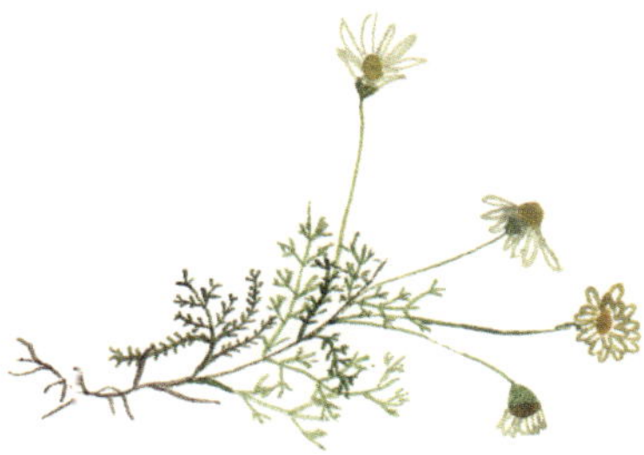

CHAMOMILE

Matricaria chamomilla

When we consider comforting teas for children and adults alike, we think of chamomile. The pretty little white and yellow flowers turn tea bright yellow and soothe us. In homeopathy, chamomile is considered "for babies of any age." Drinking incredible, picked-same-year chamomile tea will forever turn you off to the dust that is found in tea bags, and when I have amazing chamomile, I drink it on its own rather than blending it. But chamomile is really simple to blend, especially with other calming herbs in this category. The flowers are the part of the plant used for tea. *Matricaria*, a member of the Aster family, is so named from the Latin *matrix* (womb) and *mater* (mother). I like to think that this is because chamomile has the property of mothering, of calming down, nurturing, and providing gentle care. *Medicinal notes:* Nervine herbs like chamomile target an overactive nervous system, helping calm the body. More is more when it comes to taking nervine herbs. In order to get their full effects for medicinal value, the teas should be consumed frequently. Nervines are used as parts of comprehensive treatment plans to address anxiety, depression, and sleep issues.

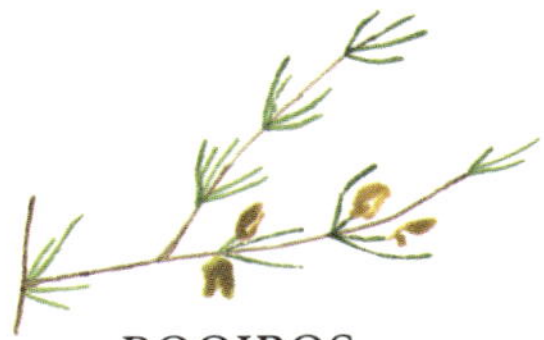

ROOIBOS

Aspalathus linearis

Native to South Africa, rooibos is sometimes called red tea for its red-orange color. Rooibos, and its close cousin, honeybush, are in the Fabaceae family. The red color and sweet flavor are created as a result of fermenting the green leaves of the plant. While some people drink the green, unfermented version, the fermented reddish-brown tea is more popular and prevalent. Because of its color and sweetness, rooibos has an uplifting, invigorating quality despite not having caffeine. Rooibos has been studied for its anti-inflammatory and antioxidant properties. Vanilla rooibos is a great blend option.

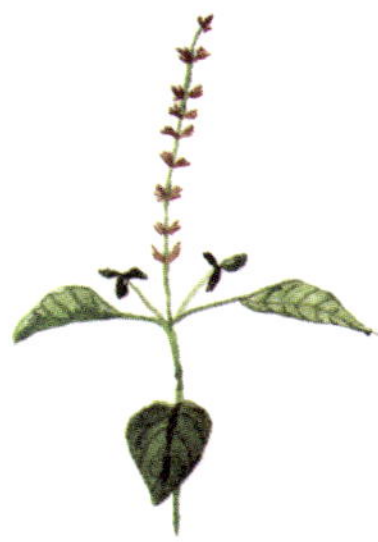

HOLY BASIL

Ocimum tenuiflorum

Holy basil, also called tulsi, was the plant that led me to study herbs. The leaf is used for tea. There are several different types of tulsi: Rama tulsi, Krishna tulsi, Amrita tulsi, and Temperate tulsi, all of which have distinct flavors. Another tulsi variety, *Ocimum Africanum,* is one of my personal favorites. The plant tends to balance our emotions and imparts a relaxed feeling overall, making it apt for any time of day. I recommend this plant to everybody. Personally, I love the flavor on its own and most often drink it that way, but uplifting plants like pine needles, cedar tips, or juniper would work well blended with it. *Medicinal notes:* Adaptogens are herbs that balance out energy levels, so they may be helpful for someone who has mood swings or struggles with fatigue. Adaptogenic teas are great because you can drink them over the course of the day without getting sleepy and also without becoming too alert.

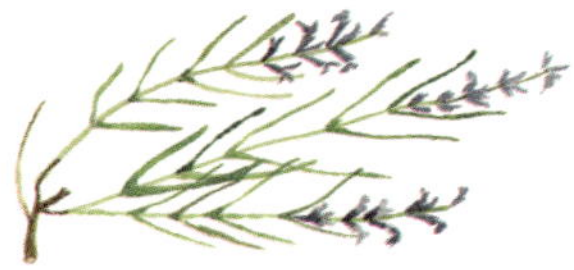

LAVENDER

Lavendula

I would love it if every person in this country woke up with lavender essential oil beside their bed and didn't speak, send an email, or do anything else until they spent three to five minutes just smelling the lavender. So many decisions are made out of hyperactivity, restlessness, anxiety, and fear. Lavender's smell, its natural purple color that is so difficult to replicate in a paint or textile, and the slightly bitter flavor of the flowers make it a natural addition to evening tea, bringing us steps closer to peaceful sleep. Lavender falls in the category of hypotonic herbs, specifically aiding in sleep. It is easy to blend with other herbs for sleep, such as California poppy and lemon balm.

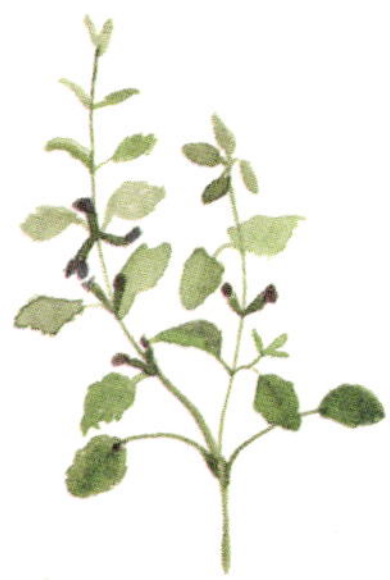

LEMON BALM

Melissa officinalis

A member of the mint family, lemon balm is slightly sour, aromatic, and a little sweet. It's a wonderful plant for stressed-out city people. As an entryway into calming plants, I prefer it to chamomile because it has a more accessible flavor. You can prepare tea from the leaves of the fresh or dried herb and it's delightful both on its own or blended. It can be a good complement to herbs that are slightly bitter to balance out the taste, and also as an accompaniment to chamomile and other flowers. *Medicinal notes:* Lemon balm is used in antidepressant blends. Keep in mind that some of the other herbs in this category, like St. John's Wort, can interact with pharmaceutical antidepressants so they shouldn't be taken in conjunction.

-five-

Romantic

"Love and scandal are the best sweeteners of tea."
—Henry Fielding, *Love in Several Masques* (1728)

I chose the plants in this section based on their seductive quality. Some for an alluring, intoxicating smell, overlapping with the perfume and fragrance world; others for their mysterious history and lore. Romance is a vital part of being alive, and I believe that striving to incorporate components of it, including beauty, art, and mystery, every day, makes life more meaningful and helps us reconnect with ourselves, our partners, and our loved ones.

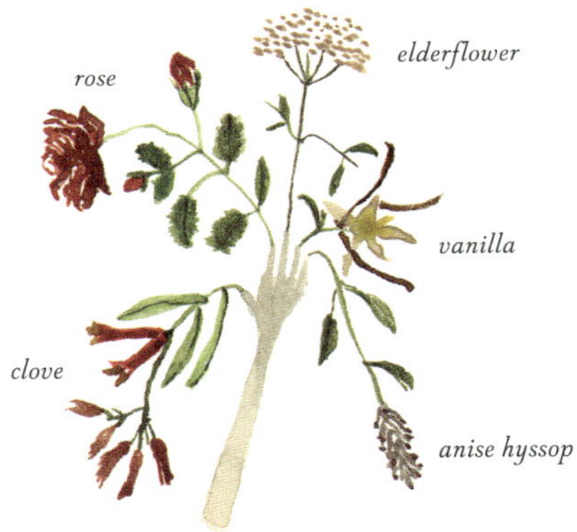

ANISE HYSSOP

Agastache foeniculum

Anise hyssop stands out in the mint family for its soft fennel flavor. The leaves, stem, and purple flower are all used in tea, so there are small lilac-colored dots that make the tea even more lovely. Largely absent from the herbal literature, anise tastes soothing, uplifting, and has a suggestion of that menthol feeling that peppermint has, without actually tasting minty. This tea is so refreshing iced and creates a lovely pale-green iced tea. Anise hyssop stands strong on its own, but I blend it with roses and cedar in the Masha Tea Love blend. I would consider blending it with other flowers as I think it makes a strong base note. Pair it with fennel seed to highlight that flavor but still bring the herbal backdrop of the mint family.

CLOVE

Syzygium aromaticum

Clove comes from a dried flower bud originally native to Indonesia. The smell of clove may be considered ambrosial. Perfumers pair it with notes like tobacco, vanilla, nutmeg, and ginger. For tea, consider it with aromatic spices like cinnamon and cardamom, balanced with black tea. Because it is high in essential oils, a clove's scent will make a stronger impression than its flavor, so a little bit goes a long way for that purpose. Clove has been studied for its antimicrobial properties. A component of clove, eugenol, has been used in dentistry, and clove, like mint, is a common flavoring in toothpastes and other dental hygiene products.

ELDERBERRY

Sambucus nigra

Previously classified in the same family as honeysuckle (Caprifoliaceae), elderberries have since been reclassified into the Viburnaceae family. While all parts of the tree, including bark, root, and stem, have a medicinal or functional use—the berries, in particular, are often made into elderberry syrup as a support during cold and flu season. For tea, I focus specifically on the delicate and gentle elderflowers. I pair elderflower with other garden herbs, like mint, lavender, or nettle, but as I mentioned previously, I was inspired by a turmeric-elderflower blend. The sweetness of the elderflower complements the mild aroma of the turmeric. That blend has made me consider elderberry as a way to add a sweet floral note to blends. *Medicinal notes:* Elderberry is often used for its antiviral properties. Antimicrobial herbs include antibacterial, antiviral (as in this case), antiparasitic, and antifungal preparations. These should mostly be taken under the care of an experienced practitioner to treat a specific illness.

ROSE

Rosa spp.

"If Zeus chose us a King of the flowers in his mirth,
He would call to the rose, and would royally crown it."
—Sappho, "Song of the Rose" (ca. 600 BCE)

Along with roses, plants in the Rosacea family include apples, quince, plums, pears, cherries, and almonds. Romantic fruits. Apricots, peaches, strawberries, blackberries, and raspberries are all in this family as well. If you think about the blossoms on these fruits, you see why. Beyond the smell and the delicate petals, and all of the poetry around roses, I think that the lusciousness of this family as a whole helps communicate the romance of roses. For tea, the dry petals—or whole rose buds and rose hips (the seed pods)—are of interest. The rose hips are full of vitamin C, flavonoids, and other nutrients, and are often made into jams as well as teas. They have a tart flavor with a touch of sweetness. Rose petals, in contrast, prove more aromatic than flavorful. I include them in blends for their smell, color, and beauty. Rose tea on its own is quite mild. With aromatic plants, often the smell comes in the oil, and because oil is not soluble in water, it's difficult to extract the flavor in tea. That shouldn't deter you from using these types of plants: smell is a powerful component of tea. I blend roses with many herbs—anise hyssop, holy basil, cedar, black tea. Any tea that can give it a platform to shine and will complement versus overpower its smell.

VANILLA

Vanilla planifolia

When we drink vanilla tea, or cook with vanilla, we use the fruit of an orchid. *Vanilla planifolia* is one of the few orchids that produces edible fruit. Make sure to get plump, well-stored vanilla beans for home use. I use half a bean for a large cup of tea, which I enjoy on its own. Halve the vanilla bean, then slice it up and put it in water. Bring the water to a boil with the sliced vanilla to make a rich tea. It can be interesting blended with clove, cinnamon, and other warming spices.

-six-

Resilient

Many of the plants in this section are considered weeds that you'd find growing wild near creeks or meadows, or even on the edges of city sidewalks. I consider that a testament to their resilience and strength.

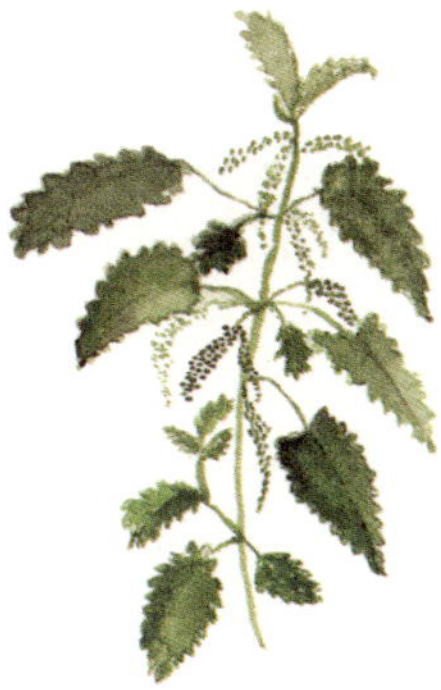

NETTLE

Urtica dioica

Stinging nettle is fittingly called *Urtica*. Urticaria refers to hives, and if you touch fresh stinging nettle, it will sting you and cause a hive-like rash. Even dried nettle will sting and make your skin red, painful, and itchy. Luckily, for our purposes, that property goes away with cooking (nettle pesto is really great), heating (broths and soups), or pouring hot water over it for tea. When handling fresh nettle, or dried whole leaves, you must wear gloves. For tea, we brew the leaves and root. I drank nettle tea during and after my pregnancy. My midwife's clinic was called Nettle Wellness for good reason—nettle is one of the most common herbs used in women's health. I like to make infusions of nettle so that I can drink it over the course of the day (refer to cold-brew recipe, page 94). This can be made with fresh or dried herbs. Nettle can be enjoyed throughout the day, much like water, because it has a fresh, wholesome flavor, and tastes nutritious, due in part to its abundance of calcium, magnesium, potassium, iron, and other nutrients. As a blend, it pairs well with other nourishing herbs like burdock and echinacea.

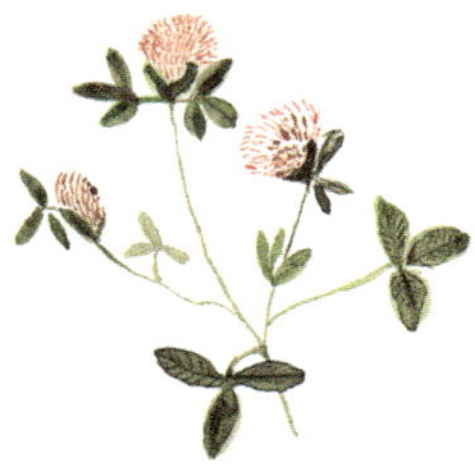

RED CLOVER

Trifolium pretense

I remember picking red clover as a child. It dots fields of grass in the countryside and abandoned lots along the sides of highways. The flowers, both because of their round shape and dark pink color, make for a lovely addition to tea. The flavor of the flowers is slightly sweet, and it doesn't have a strong accompanying floral scent, so it's a lovely way to make a tea look floral without imparting that flavor profile. In truth, the taste is relatively mild. *Medicinal notes:* Red clover is used in blends that support the upper respiratory system. I also use it in blends for women's health and for new moms, paired with raspberry leaf and nettle.

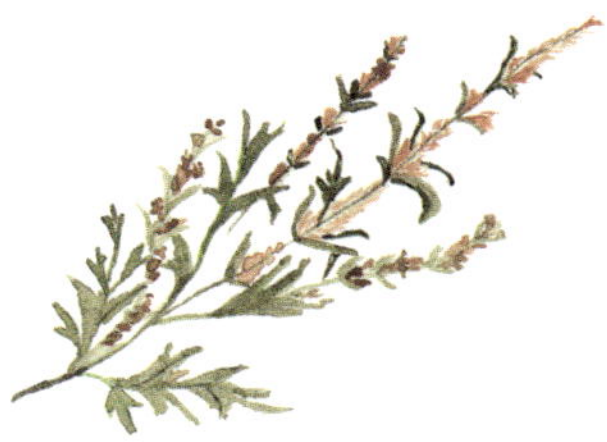

MUGWORT

Artemisia vulgaris

Mugwort is one of my favorite plants to see growing around New York City. In late summer and early fall, it's everywhere, which is interesting because its lore is that it's used to help you remember your dreams (a perfect match for a city of dreamers). Its relatives are in the Asteracea (daisy) family, the same as echinacea. Mugwort can be distinguished in the wild by having white underneath the leaves, and having pointed versus blunt leaf segments. The tea is made of the leaves which, flavorwise, can be a touch bitter. It is otherwise pretty herbal and earthy tasting. Because of its slight bitterness, a property that it shares with the tea plant, it was used as a substitute for tea in England for those who couldn't afford black tea.

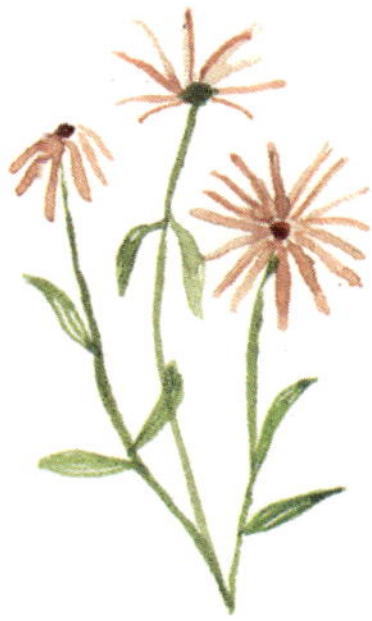

ECHINACEA

Echinacea

You've seen echinacea growing in ornamental gardens, the long, thin flowers in pinks, whites, and purples with little cone seed pods in the middle. Echinacea root is often used in tea, though the stems and flowers can be included, too. Commonly found in immune-supportive blends, or in respiratory support alongside mullein or marshmallow, I like to include it in teas for its grassy earthiness. Echinacea, a member of the Asteracea (daisy) family, is one of the most popular and widely used herbal remedies. Since so many people drink tea from tea bags, people forget that teas are plants that grow in soil, subject to the elements of water and sunshine and the people who harvest, pick, and dry them. With echinacea, you remember the soil due to its flavor, so I use the plant in blends where I want to evoke that memory. For Masha Tea, I created a blend called Earth Tea that includes echinacea, burdock root, and calendula flowers, which makes you think about the parts of a whole plant—root, stem, and flower.

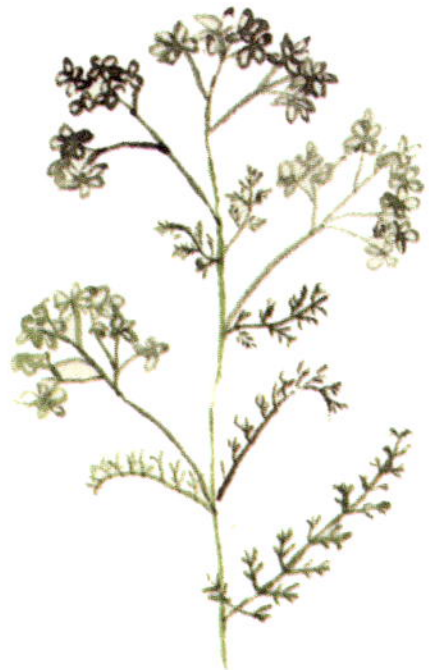

YARROW

Achillea millefolium

Of all the plants described, yarrow tastes the most "medicinal," meaning bitter. I'll admit that I prefer to pick it for flower arrangements or to use it in tincture form, but I do want to describe it because maybe you'll fall in love with it in your own way. *Achillea* is named for the Greek god Achilles—he used the plant to heal his wounds. Yarrow, along with a plant called Devil's Club, are used for energetic protection and boundaries. In the past, I've taken a few drops of the tincture before going into stressful situations. The way to think about this doesn't have to be literal—it doesn't mean that yarrow will help you be better about boundaries—but what it does mean is that you've taken a moment to pause before a difficult situation to bring intentionality to it, and maybe to contemplate what you can do to make it easier. I would use just a bit in tea because of the bitterness and consider it as a digestif before or after a heavy meal. Another use for yarrow is in a decongestant blend to help decrease swelling in the upper respiratory tract.

Blending Teas

Once you start to collect teas and herbs, you will want to blend teas—you won't be able to help yourself. Of course, you'll first have to drink and enjoy the teas on their own to decide which blends to make. Some herbs are more effective, and even taste better, when mixed with others. Take rose tea. Unless there is some artificial flavoring, the taste is so subtle. If you still want to experience the beauty and smell of rose while really enjoying a cup of tea, roses are beautiful to mix with other teas, herbs, or flowers. On the other end, if you're wanting to drink something like California poppy, which can be quite bitter, combining it with something sweet like licorice or anise hyssop can take the edge off of the bitterness. In naturopathic medicine, even medicinal herbal blends should taste good to the person taking them. Reasons to blend teas can be medicinal, for enhancing flavor or beauty, or just be for fun and experimentation. All reasons are justified. Blending tea just means mixing at least two different types of herbs together, keeping in mind flavor, color, aesthetics, and scent.

Flavor

If blending tea for flavor, it's important to first understand each tea on its own, starting with how long it takes for the flavor to come through; for example, with green tea, you can drink it after just a minute of brewing. As a general rule, you can taste tea leaves quite quickly, whereas roots and seeds take longer to brew. Teas that take different lengths of time make interesting blends, because the flavor changes dramatically depending on when you drink it. This is something that can be enjoyed by drinking a pot of tea from small cups. Refilling the cups as you go allows you to taste the teas at different brewing stages.

The flavor of tea is different from flavor*ing*. Commercial flavoring is often done in large blending drums with perfumes, additives, or essential oils. Although blending and scenting teas can add an additional dimension to tea, the process may also sometimes be used to obscure the quality of substandard teas.

Color

Tea is a visual delight. Aside from the beauty of teaware and accoutrements, there's the color of tea itself. One way to approach choosing tea is similar to choosing a wardrobe or an outfit for the day: instead of thinking about what color you want to wear, think about what color you want to feel in your body.

GREEN

matcha, green tea, mint, the leaves of herbs

Is green the most opulent color? When I think of it in terms of green clothes, I first think of hikingwear, but there is the other side of green—the rich, jewel-tone version, which tells a different story. There's the rich green of velvet furniture and feeling green with envy, street-sign green, a green traffic light.

RED

hibiscus, rooibos, roses

A color of strength, power, urgency, intensity, red teas are a favorite to make for guests for the effect of the color. The color of hibiscus is matched by its bright tartness. Rose buds in tea can similarly be considered; the visual effect is more striking than for the flavor they provide—which is typically quite subtle. The same goes for red hues of pink and purple, with flowers like cherry blossoms and lavender.

BROWN

black tea, roots

The color of soil and earth, brown, from amber to chocolate tones, suggests richness and depth. When tea is brown, there is a suggestion of bitterness.

YELLOW

chamomile, calendula, chrysanthemum

Yellow suggests calm, friendliness, ease. The color yellow is related to the liver, and bile, and so liver-supportive herbs that improve digestion and detoxification may be classified here.

Aesthetic Considerations

Tea should be beautiful—a sensory experience that layers flavor with smell, the sight of the tea leaves, how they feel, and the sound of water. To make a blend look or smell even more is reason enough to introduce a component to a blend.

Scent

Though closely related, scent and taste are distinct senses. You first taste tea with your nose. When blending tea, it's okay to layer flowers and plants into teas for the smell alone, even if they don't add much to the flavor profile.

Ratios

A blend of equal parts of three different herbs is a lot different than a blend with a lot of one herb and a little bit of some others. The art of tea blending involves intentionality around these ratios. Remember that blending tea is not a science and you can experiment with blends to see what you like best. If you use herbs that you like and know how to brew on their own, you can't go wrong. Unless I'm making chai, which can include many different herbs, I like to keep blends very simple and use only two or three herbs.

One thing to remember with different herbs is that a tablespoon of black tea, for example, does not weigh the same as a tablespoon of fennel. So, using the example blend of black, chamomile, and fennel, if you put in a tablespoon of each, the fennel will be heaviest, black tea will be in the middle, and chamomile will be lightest. If you are somebody who likes to reproduce a recipe exactly, you can eye it the first time but still jot down the weights and amounts as you go.

Medicinal Herbal Blends

One reason to blend teas is to make a personalized medicinal blend for yourself. You might want to compound the power of healing teas by mixing them together; for example, if you're having trouble sleeping because you can't calm down at night, you could blend several teas from the calming category (see page 191). Maybe you're having trouble sleeping, and you're also overcoming a winter cold. Then you might blend teas from the calming category and also include one or two warming herbs into that blend. Continuing with this concept, maybe you're overcoming a cold, and so you're using warming herbs, but you also know that there are herbs in the romantic category, like elderberry, that have antimicrobial properties. Those might be good to include in the blend. Finally, when it comes to medicinal herbs, sometimes you might want to make blends to mask the flavor of an herb that you want to include for medicinal value but whose taste you don't really like.

Based on your short-term healing needs, choose teas or categories you might be interested in, get them for home, and try them (if you're having recurring health issues, medicinal use of herbs should be in conjunction with the care of a licensed medical provider). In addition to their healing properties, also notice which ones you are attracted to visually, smell good to you, and that you taste and simply want more of. Especially if those align with your healing goals, and they often will, drink more of those teas. To me, healing means feeling freer in our bodies and day-to-day. Feeling more at ease, feeling well. With teas and herbs, different people crave different plants, so try to find the ones that speak to you.

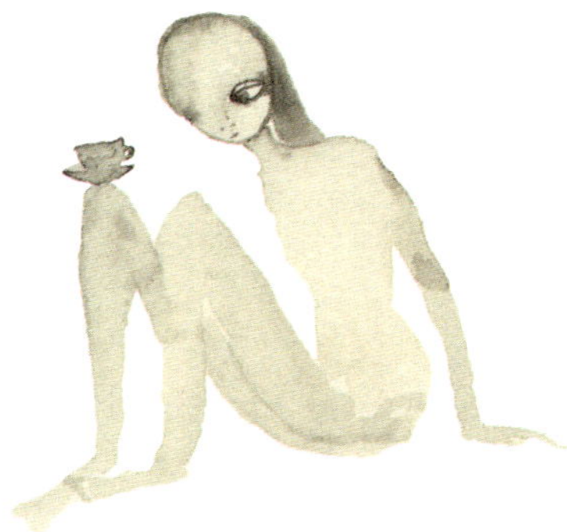

Women's Health

Herbs used for women's health issues can often be considered in terms of cycles. That can mean period cycles, but it can also pertain to cycles of life. Different herbs support fertility, pregnancy, postpartum, and the transition into menopause. There are ways to use herbs for specific conditions—like using high-dose viburnum (colloquially called cramp bark) and ginger for period pain, or using sage to help with hot flashes in perimenopause, but even then, a holistic approach would include addressing imbalances in the cycle overall, not only treating pain.

Pregnancy and Postpartum

Tea can be so soothing for all phases of fertility—conception, pregnancy, and postpartum. Establishing a ritual can be a lot simpler for parents-to-be who have more freedom to take the whole morning or evening to themselves.

When thinking about teas for fertility, anything that helps keep your stress levels low is best, so the nervine category of herbs would be a great consideration. Once I got pregnant, I developed a rhythm with my teas. I never stopped drinking caffeine, but I lost the taste for coffee (aversions to flavors are common in pregnancy), and I shifted over to having a cup of black tea with milk and honey every morning. Throughout the day, I drank a lot of nettle tea. At the time, I had some grown locally on a small farm on Long Island, and I drank pure nettle tea every day. It made my body feel nourished—I just loved it. On that note, pregnant women are constantly being told what to do: what to put in their bodies, what not to put in their bodies, how much to put in their bodies, and so on. Yet they are never told to follow their intuition and to listen to what their bodies are telling them.

From a naturopathic perspective, there are many supportive exercises and foods to optimize a pregnancy, but the focus here will be on tea.

The two most soothing herbs for pregnancy are nettle and red raspberry leaf, enjoyed either hot or as a cold infusion (see Herbal Infusions, page 92). Nettle, fresh or dried, is high in chlorophyll, vitamins A, C, D, and K, calcium, potassium, and iron. Red raspberry leaf is rich in vitamin E and C, calcium, and iron, and contains an alkaloid called fragrine, which tonifies the pelvic region. A beautiful tea for pregnancy would be either one of these herbs or mixing them together in equal parts. Another way to enjoy them is to alternate them weekly.

Many women suffer from reflux during pregnancy, and mint can exacerbate the condition, so I would choose something other than peppermint for those experiencing reflux. Fennel tea is a lovely alternative, as it has a soothing effect on the digestive system. Another herb to keep in the rotation for pregnancy is fresh ginger, which can help with nausea. Finally, I love chamomile and lemon balm tea as soothing options to signal the body and nervous system to calm down.

To prepare for childbirth, most people pack the essentials in their hospital bag, but this is an opportunity to bring some luxury into an otherwise sterile experience. Things like herbal soap for the bathroom, tea, beautiful teacups to properly drink tea after the birth, local honey, and lemons. In addition to using lemons for tea after birth, they're also lovely for aromatherapy during labor—I literally held them like stress balls and brought them to my nose to smell them.

Postpartum, also called "the Fourth Trimester," starts with the three to six months after pregnancy. Tea can be a really special aspect of postpartum life, which is marked by love, recovery, and making space for a new person. Consider a blend including red clover, red raspberry leaf, and nettle, which can soothe the postpartum body.

Chamomile and lemon balm are lovely for keeping mood stable. For breastfeeding moms, fennel tea is an example of a galactagogue, an herb that helps promote milk supply; on the other side, sage tea can slow it down for those who are oversupplying. Echinacea, with its effects on the immune system, makes a great base for a postpartum tea to help support the overall health of the new mother. Personally, I drank a lot of holy basil tea postpartum. I love the way that it makes me feel—centered, at ease, like myself—but I also love the way it tastes.

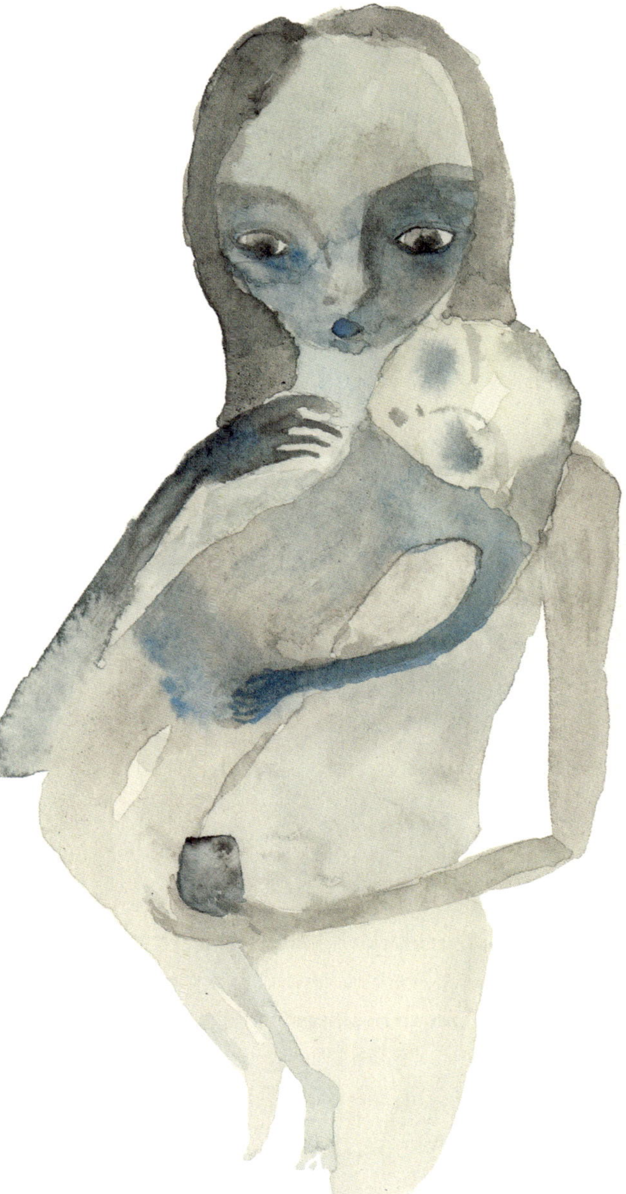

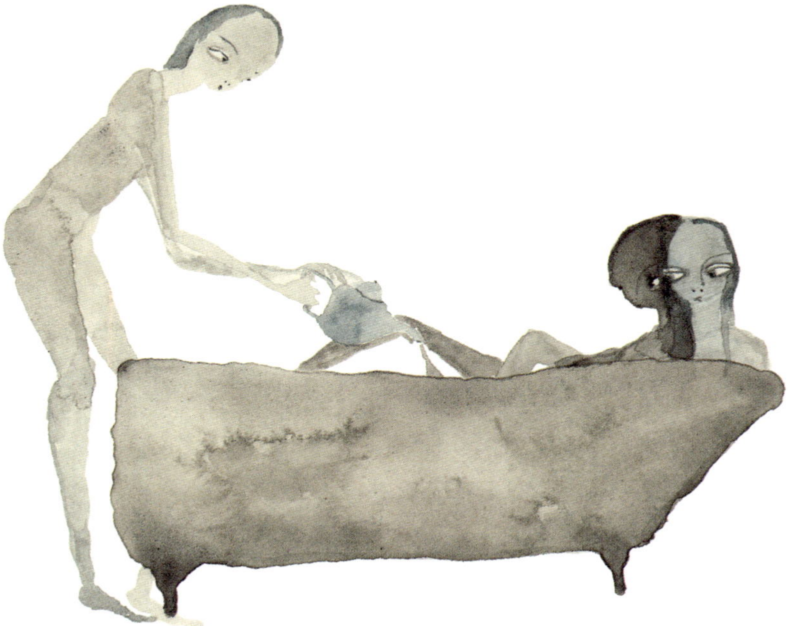

"Beauty (was) a gift which, in the eyes of New York,
justified every success, and excused
a certain number of failings."
—Edith Wharton,
The Age of Innocence (1920)

– 13 –

Tea and Beauty

Tea plays a role in beauty rituals—not only through drinking tea, but also by using different types of teas and herbs to create beauty routines, skincare products, and luxurious self-care treatments.

I consider these rituals for everyday self-care—sunscreen, time for a relaxing bath, face oil—but also for the more luxurious, or spaced-out upkeep—the sauna, a facial steam. When it comes to the relationship between tea and beauty rituals, keep a couple of factors in mind: First, use tea as a part of an experience—like a cup of hormone-balancing licorice tea before a massage or a facial, or antioxidant-rich green tea after the sauna—and second, use tea and herbs themselves as part of skincare and beauty rituals.

When it comes to caring for our skin and bodies, what goes in (nutrition, hydration, what we read, listen to, the media we consume) is as important as what goes on (creams, sunlight, soaps or cleansers during a shower). In the case of tea, the adage "only put on your body what you would put in your body" rings true, as herbs that we drink as teas can also often be used as topical skincare products.

In this chapter, we'll explore best practices for skin health, and I'll provide instructions for using tea in easy beauty applications and incorporating tea in meditation rituals.

How to Make a Tea Bath

A perfect bath to me is in the bright light on a Sunday afternoon, listening to music with a pot of tea beside me, and a magazine, folded in half, a little wet from the bath water. An afternoon bath is a sign of freedom—nowhere to be, no one to answer to, the luxury of time. The sense of freedom—escaping from the pressures of schedules, responsibility, and time constraints—is such a key aspect of wellness that is often overlooked. At its best, an unstructured afternoon in the bath can accomplish that. I started making Bath Flowers for Masha Tea to ease the experience of an at-home tea bath. Below are some plants that I like to use. If you don't have access to tea or flowers, you can use the essential oils, though the whole plant is preferable because you get the visual experience as well. If you have access to fresh, organic herbs and flowers, use those instead of the dried ones. There is nothing more beautiful or fragrant.

As the tub fills with water, add a couple of pumps of your preferred soap. Add in 2 cups (475 g) Epsom salts, which have a high magnesium content thus relaxing your muscles, as the tub fills for the most calming results.

ADD HERBS AND FLOWERS:

Mix and match from these options.

HIBISCUS: Use a generous 2 to 3 cups (about 50 to 100 g) whole hibiscus flowers to turn the bath a bright pink color. (If you use more hibiscus than any other herb, the pink color will be more prevalent than any other color.)

GREEN TEA: Use 1 cup (40 to 50 g) green tea to turn the bath a lovely mint green color and to benefit from the restorative properties of green tea for skin.

CALENDULA FLOWERS: Use 1 cup (about 10 to 15 g) calendula flowers to sooth irritated skin and to enjoy the petals brushing up against you.

(recipe continues)

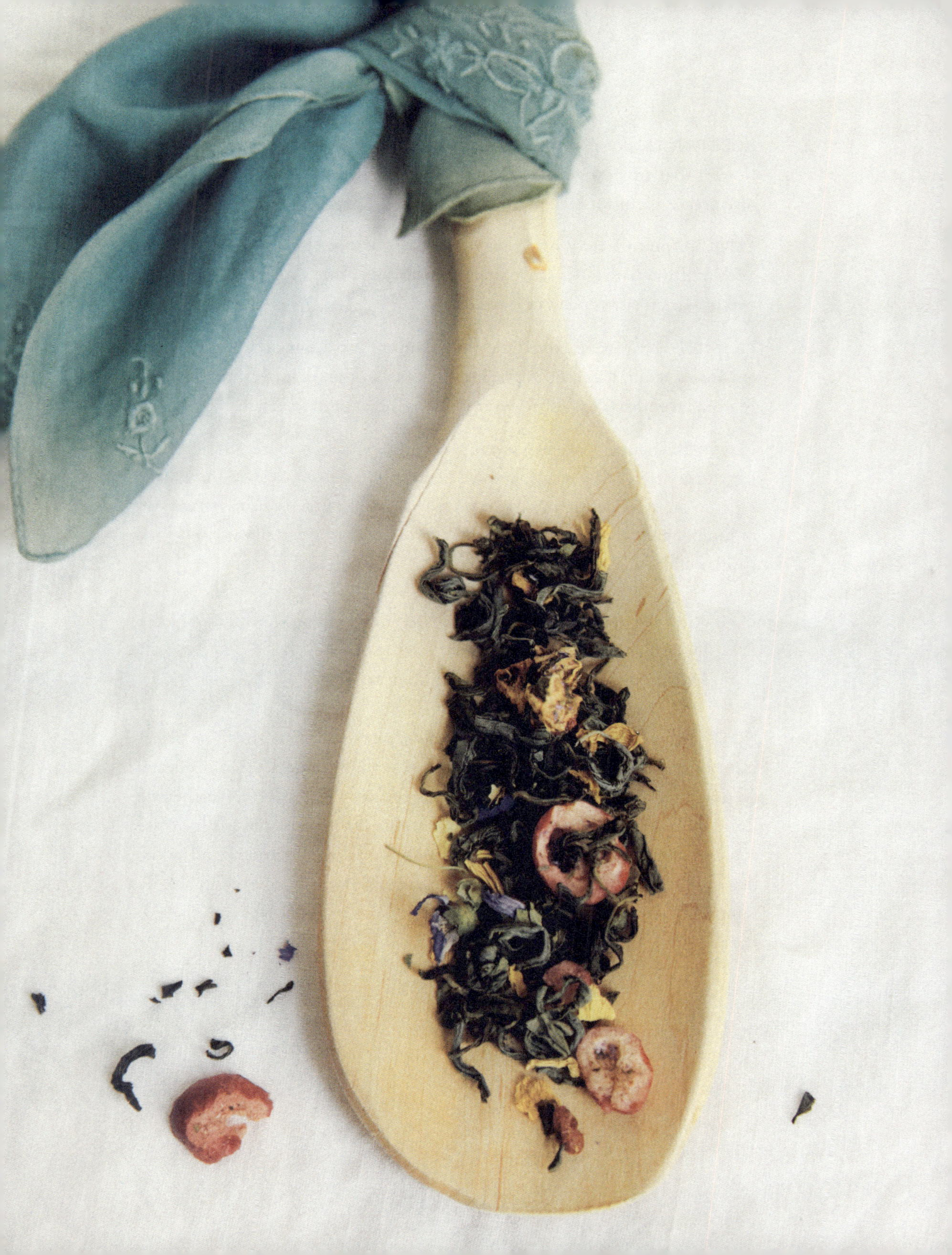

ROSE PETALS: For pure romance, use a dozen fresh roses (make sure to get flowers that are pesticide-free). Two to 3 cups (10 to 30 g) dried rose petals also create a feminine, romantic effect.

CITRUS: You can use 2 or 3 sliced lemons or oranges for an abundant, fun, and uplifting bath. I also love including citrus in baths for children, or you can use dried citrus peels or essential oils.

LAVENDER: It can be incredible for a calming bath but because the flowers are so small, it can be very difficult to clean the tub afterward. For this reason, lavender is easiest when thrown in the bath in a sachet.

CEDAR: It creates a subtle, woodsy aroma, which is incredibly grounding. I use dried cedar tips that have been snipped from trees in the Pacific Northwest, so the clippings themselves look like tiny trees. Pine, spruce, fir, or juniper can all be used in its place. Also consider linden flower pods for a similar effect. Use 2 or 3 handfuls.

After the bath, drain the tub and rinse the floral residue off (see Note).
Dry off and remove the flowers from the bath.
Moisturize your skin with a body oil or serum.

NOTE: When you are putting whole herbs and/or flowers, fresh or dried, into the bath, you have to thoroughly clean the residue so that it doesn't go down the drain and clog up the tub. I consider this effort a worthwhile trade-off for being able to touch and interact with the plants while you're soaking. If this is truly off-putting to you, get muslin bags and put all of the herbs, flowers, or citrus that you want to use in the bag so you can simply remove it after the bath.

How to Make an Herbal Steam

The purpose of a facial steam is to open up the pores in the face, bringing blood flow to the area. Outside of beauty rituals, facial steams can feel great during sinus infections or upper respiratory tract infections because they open the airways and stimulate the circulatory system. You can use fresh herbs, dry herbs, or a combination of the two in the hot water when you are preparing your steam. Exercise the utmost care in your setup, as you are putting your face very close to extremely hot water. Be sure not to touch the water *with any body part*. Be sure your face is clean and dry.

Bring a pot of water to a boil. Meanwhile, prepare an ice bath and place a towel in it. When the water boils, add in 2 tablespoons of herbs and/or flowers. (See Choosing Herbs for Steams below to select herbs for your steam.) Simmer for 2 to 3 minutes and then carefully pour the hot water into a large bowl on the table you will sit by.

Put your face over the bowl and cover both your head and the bowl with a dry towel, so that steam is created between the bowl and your face and is insulated by the towel. It gets really hot in there so open up the towel to allow air in as needed or come out occasionally to catch a breath. Ideally, steam a total of 8 to 10 minutes, inclusive of the breaks.

After a steam, pat your face dry, squeeze out the towel soaking in the cold water, and apply it to your face. Your open pores and clean face make it a perfect time for a nourishing skin care routine. The optimal step after an herbal steam would be a face mask (see page 215).

Choosing Herbs for Steams

HERBS FOR RADIANT SKIN: Use herbs that you have on hand and that smell nice to you. Comfrey, calendula, and chamomile are always great base herbs.

HERBS FOR NORMAL TO OILY SKIN: Sage and rosemary can be slightly drying, so include them with or in place of the comfrey, calendula, and chamomile or any other aromatic herbs to support oily skin.

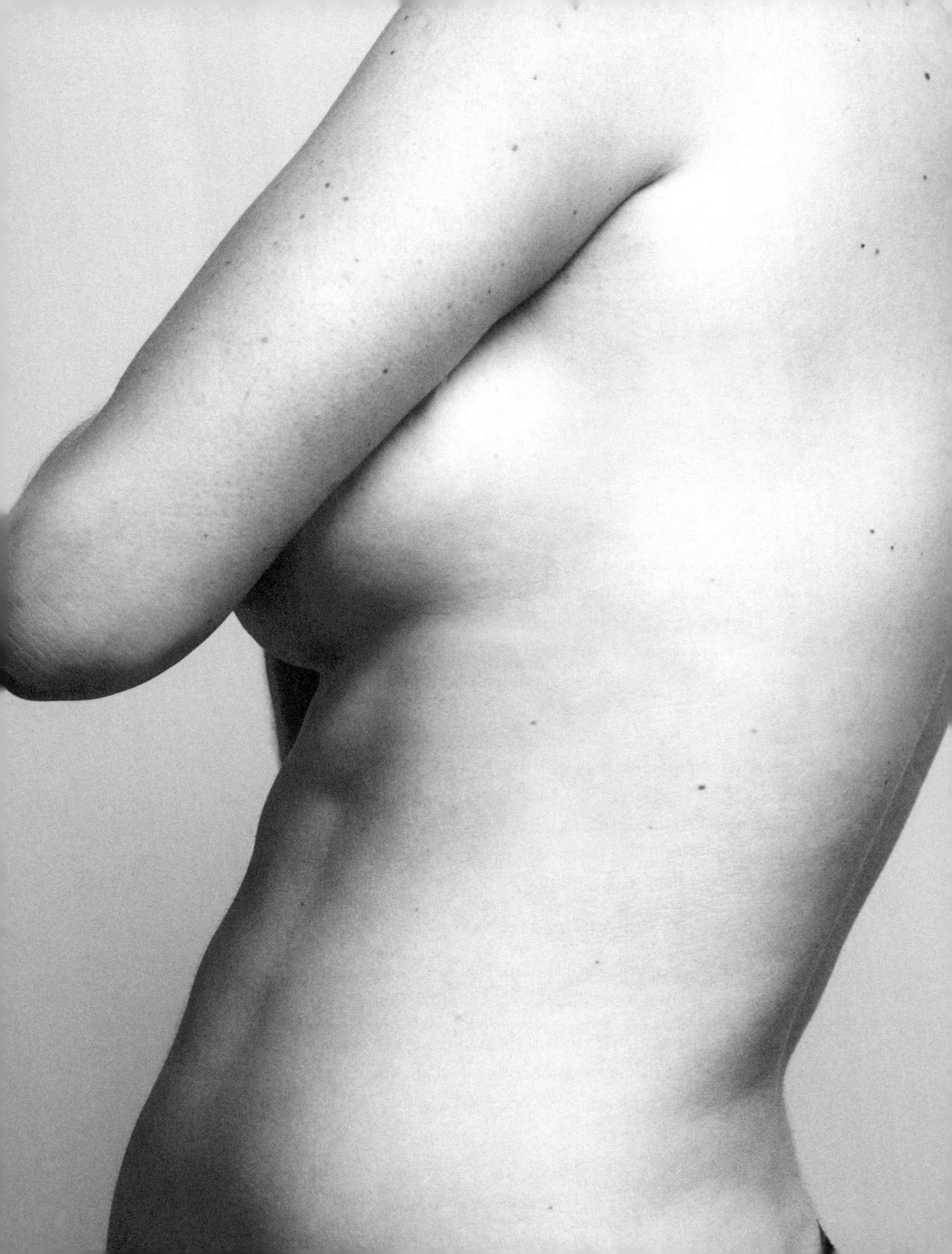

HERBS FOR NORMAL TO DRY SKIN: Rose petals and lavender can be extra hydrating. Include these with or in place of the comfrey, calendula, and chamomile or any other aromatic herbs to support dry skin.

HERBS FOR UPPER RESPIRATORY SUPPORT: For sinus infections, colds, or flus, you can use any combination of (preferably fresh) oregano, rosemary, and thyme. Oregano, rosemary, and thyme have both antiviral and antioxidant properties that make for a supportive steam in cases of sinus infections, coughs, colds, and flus.

Along with all of the herbal options above, also consider nutritive green tea and grounding conifers like spruce, pine, juniper, or cedar. You can use store-bought culinary herbs as well, or a few drops of essential oil if you don't have the herbs themselves on hand. The steam has the dual purpose of opening up your pores and using aromatherapy from the smell of the herbs to create a meditative, soothing sensation in your body.

Face Masks

I love getting facials. And at home, I aspire to be someone who does daily gua sha, a facial massage for myself, but it's a routine that I've never actually established. I prefer an at-home face mask. It's passive, energizing, and luxurious. I prefer simple recipes with minimal ingredients. The following are my go-to masks:

Honey Mask

Try to name a more heavenly match than tea and honey. I experimented with backyard beekeeping, and I find everything around bees and beekeeping so evocative, rich, and romantic. The color of gold, dripping candle wax, the language of royalty in the queen and her diet of royal jelly, the gentle hum of a honeybee on a tender pink flower.

Honey is naturally antimicrobial and therefore cleansing. Use local honey from a trusted farm or Manuka honey, as some store-bought honeys have added cane sugar or are sourced from companies that feed sugar to their bees. As a mask, honey is great for all skin types and so this mask can become part of a weekly maintenance routine. It can also feel soothing after sun damage. This mask is sticky—tie your hair back before applying—but worth it!

100 percent raw honey

Clean and dry your face. Skin should be completely dry before applying.

Pull hair back, as out of your face as possible.

Have a jar of honey dedicated to masking specifically, so that it doesn't matter that you're putting your fingers in there. Scoop a fingerful of honey from the jar and massage into your skin. Leave on for 5 to 15 minutes and wash off with warm water.

After the mask is off (and after you're out of the bath if you were in there), end with toner, and then serum or moisturizer.

NOTE: Slight redness is normal for up to 30 minutes after a mask, but it will go away.

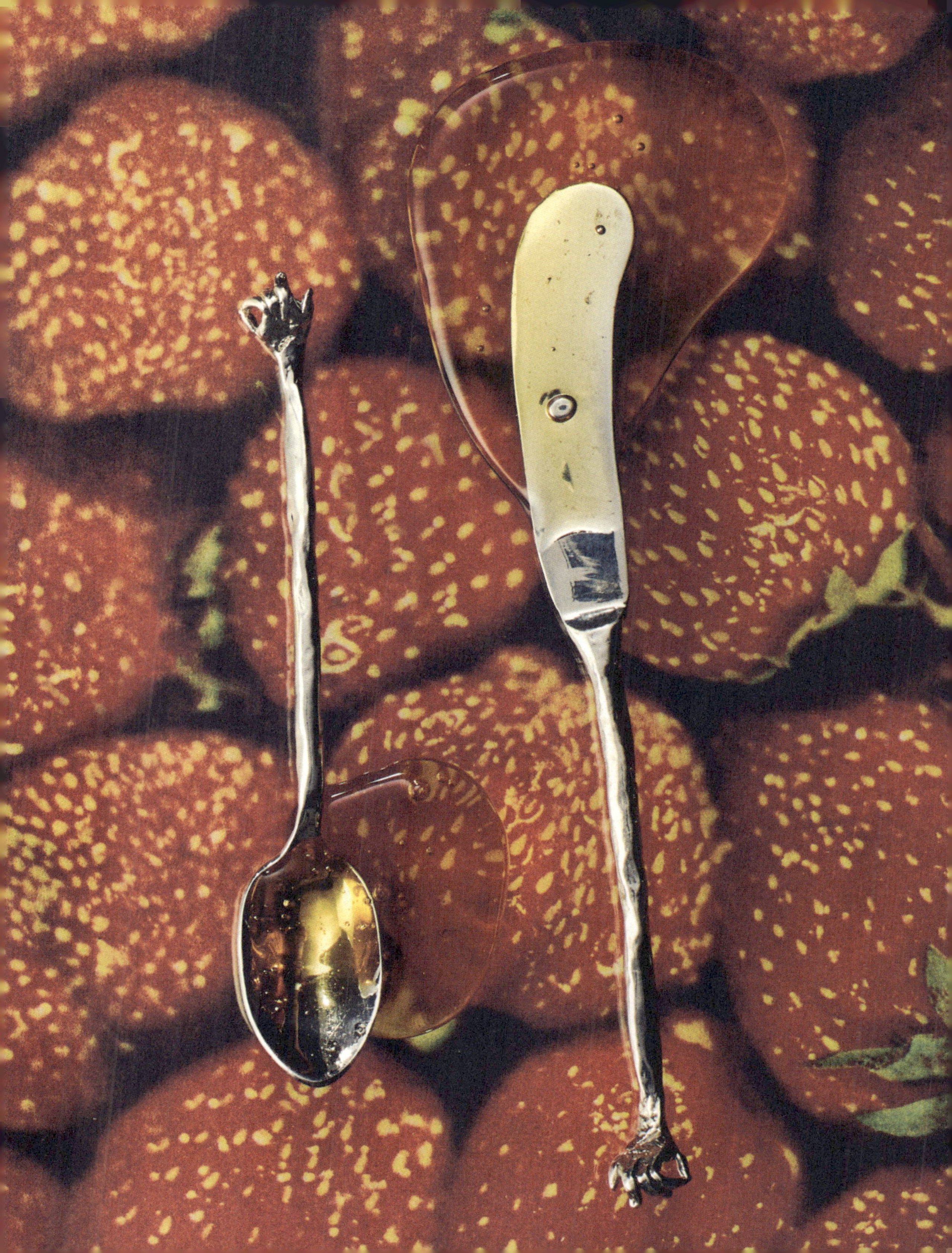

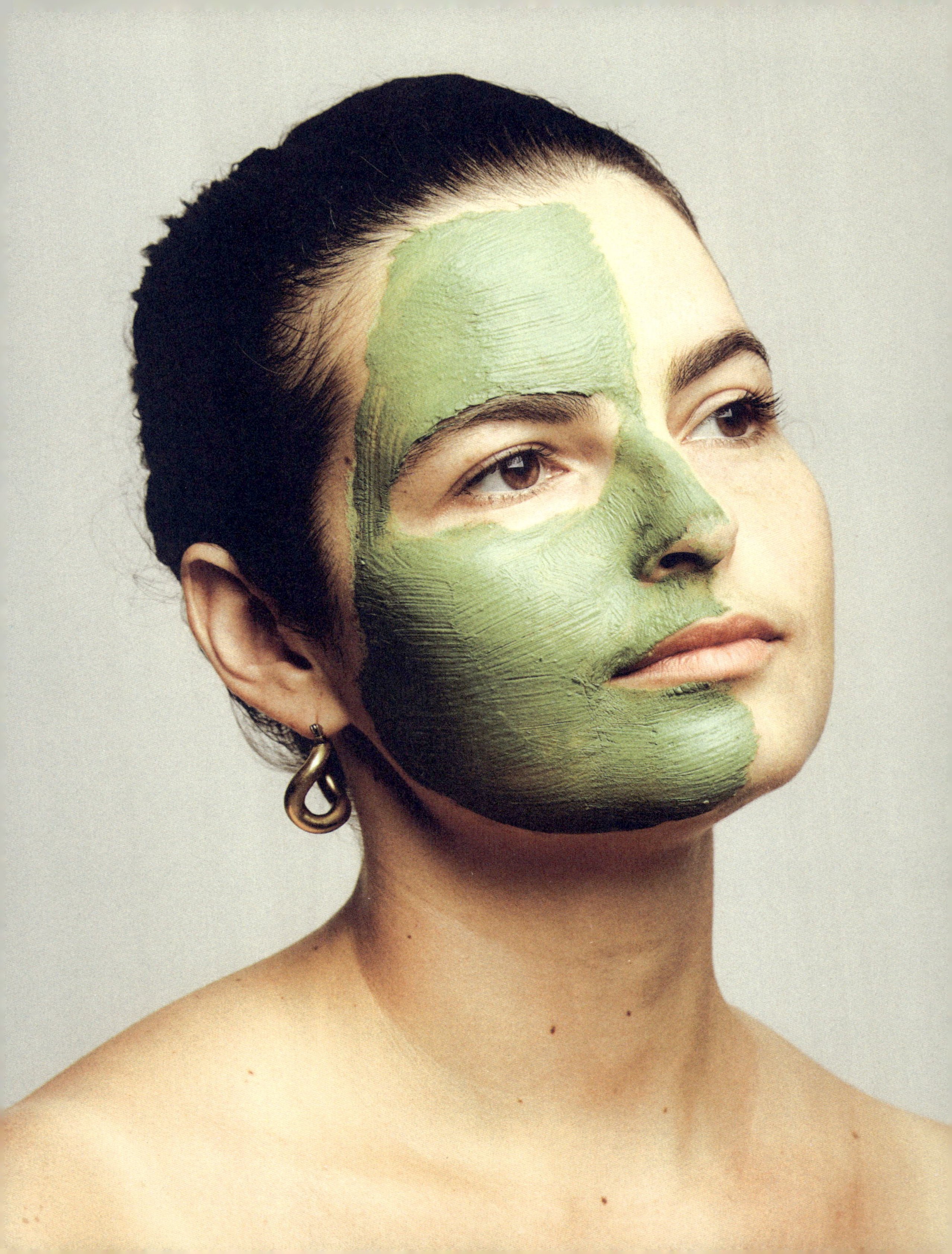

Matcha-Clay Mask

With its high antioxidant content, matcha supports healthy skin-cell turnover. Because it already comes in a powdered form, it's great combined with clay for extra support for an extracting, nutrifying mask.

2 teaspoons matcha

2 teaspoons clay (see Notes)

¼ cup (60 ml) room-temperature water

Mix equal parts matcha and clay together in a small bowl. Pour the water over the mixture and stir to combine.

Using a brush or your fingers, apply a thin layer (about ⅛-inch/3 mm thick) to face. Leave on for 15 to 20 minutes; for sensitive skin, remove after 10 to 15 minutes (leaving a mask on for too long can dry out the skin).

Remove with lukewarm water.

After a mask, apply a hydrosol or toner. Slight redness is normal for up to 30 minutes after a mask, but it will go away.

NOTES: Clay is considered detoxifying to the skin and has been used for thousands of years in beauty rituals. Clays exfoliate and cleanse the skin. These facial clays should only be used topically, on the skin, not ingested. Take care to source 100-percent pure clays. Those with reactive or sensitive skin should always try a small amount of product on the arm and leave it for 15 to 30 minutes to check for signs of irritation before doing a face mask.

THE FOLLOWING ARE A FEW CLAYS I RECOMMEND:

BENTONITE CLAY: A volcanic ash, therapeutic for clogged pores, acne, and oily skin. | FRENCH GREEN CLAY: High in sea minerals and plant matter, best for oily skin with blemishes. | RHASSOUL CLAY: Iron-rich, creating a rusty red color, best for oily, acne-prone skin. | WHITE CLAY: Stimulates circulation, most suitable for dry, sensitive skin.

Meditation and Tea

In Buddhism, tea and meditation go hand in hand, as monks aspire toward hours of uninterrupted meditation. In modern, secular life, meditation and tea can be used as tools to create a feeling of ease and calm. Meditation helps us enter the day from a clearer perspective. Because meditation decreases cortisol, it can be a tool, along with tea, for improving overall health.

It took me a long time to realize that, most simply, meditation is just breathing—but intentionally and with awareness. One way to establish a meditation ritual is to wake up early, make a cup of tea, and set aside time to do breathing exercises. If this is not possible, try four-square breathing.

I incorporate this breathing technique every day. I do it on the subway, when I'm annoyed by someone or something, and when putting my daughter to sleep—feeling that I'm quiet and calm gets her to sleep more quickly when I'm lying next to her. I've also used it while getting an MRI and during childbirth.

Breath in for four seconds.

Hold your breath for four seconds.

Breath out for four seconds.

Hold your breath for four seconds.

Repeat.

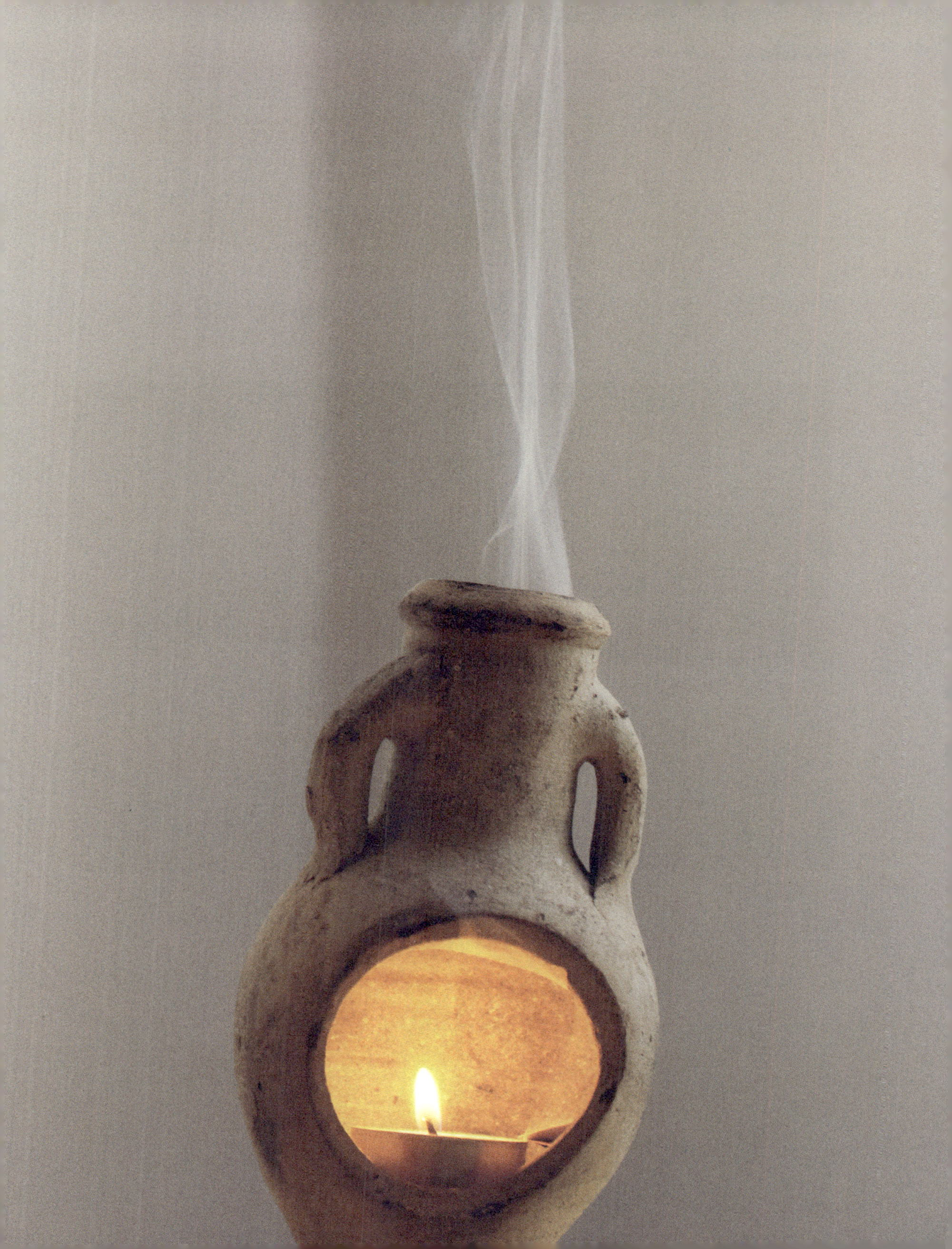

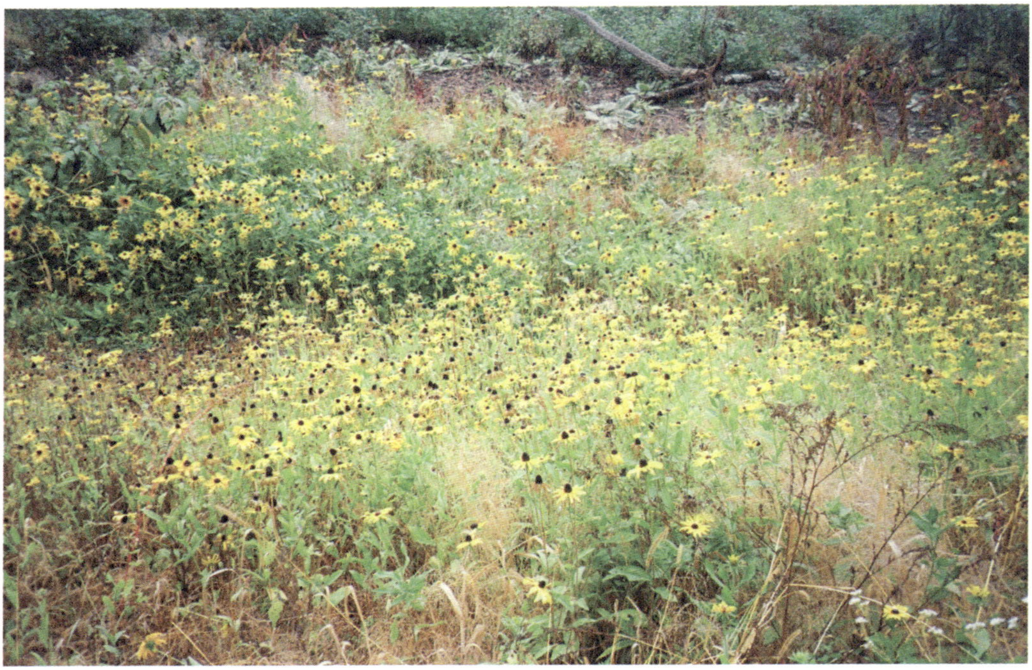

Afterword

I believe that a world in which we carve out time for tea is a more fun, chic, and peaceful place. Intentionally drinking tea can transform physical and mental well-being. Perhaps you are drinking a cup of tea as you read this, having just finished your breathing exercises, or maybe you're on a crowded subway train. I am curious about any changes in your relationship with tea culture. As for me, I'm probably listening to the birds, enjoying sunflowers, sitting high up on my fire escape with tea in hand.

Acknowledgments

I wrote most of this book at home in Brooklyn, at the Masha Tea studio, on the tea and writing retreat that I host annually in Tuscany, and in a house on a cliff in Nova Scotia, where I escaped New York's exciting distractions for quiet and solitude with my husband in late August 2025 to wring the last pages out of me.

This labor of love was made possible because so many people were kind enough to trust in the vision, and some, like my agent, Adriana Stimola, to hold my hand through it.

Much of the context for who and what made this book possible comes through in the imagery—through the stories behind the locations and pieces used in the photos. I'll share some of those stories with references to the photographs.

Photographer Fujio Emura is the kind of person you can be yourself around—always making you laugh, talented, and with a singular, conceptual perspective to his work.

Alice Waese, who painted the book's watercolors, is primarily a fine jewelry designer. Her jewelry, along with her silverware, were a delight to use in styling (pages 2, 79, 134, 217, and 226). Alice's art—her jewelry, paintings, fashion, and sensibility—are aspirational for me. I asked her immediately if she would paint for the book, and it would not be the same without her romantic, ethereal touch.

Thank you to DIOR, Lowell Hotel, and Majorelle Restaurant, where afternoon tea in Manhattan is shown on pages 17, 21, 50, and 111.

Thank you to the iconic Hotel Chelsea Spa. They offered up their penthouse balcony for our photoshoot (pages 15, 89, 137) in exchange for Masha Tea developing a custom tea blend, which we call Muse. Masha Muse Tea is now served to all spa guests.

Thank you to Ginori 1735, for the gorgeous teaware (pages 2, 10, 15, 55, 69, 124, 131, 148, and 226) and to Natalia Criado for her plates (pages 79 and 124).

Outside of the hotels, Fujio and I shot in my apartment, around my Greenpoint neighborhood, and in his studio. Stylist Rebecca Bartoshesky worked with us on the studio images (pages 10, 70, 73, 74, 79, 80, 85, 86, 95, 96, 101, 117, 124, 134, 140, 142, 144, 148, 153, and 217).

Several pieces were gifted to me by Linda Rizzo—the plates on pages 15 and 120, and the Hermès scarf on page 47—which, outside of the book, have become staples in my life and wardrobe.

I used my grandfather's cups while wearing Ahlem sunglasses in the shot on the street on page 18. Fujio and I drank so much licorice tea that day.

Some of my 35mm travel images were also included—from Masha Tea sourcing trips and from writing trips for my Tea Lover's Guide series for *Vogue*: Azuma tea farm in Uji, Japan (page 28), Naturalitea farm in Shizuoka, Japan (page 37), Maraviglia Olive Oil Farm in Tuscany (page 41), the forest near Eugene, Oregon (page 42), my sister at hotel Portrait Milano (page 56), Trunk House Hotel in Tokyo (page 59), probably the best hotel experience I've ever had, wild rose tea from an Akihiro Nikaido cup (page 93), black-eyed Susans in the Hudson Valley at Troutbeck (page 222).

In terms of handmade ceramics, Shino Takeda's bowl with kintsugi by Yuki Gunji is shown on page 73. The cover photo shows a vintage cup I sourced in Milan that shattered on its flight home to New York; Miwa Neishi repaired it with kintsugi. Asia Sosnowski's pottery is seen on pages 80, 86, and 124.

Family pieces were incorporated throughout the book: We used a glass that my dad bought in Prague as a gift for his parents for the matcha shot on page 101; my husband's great-grandmother's milk saucer is seen on pages 120 and 137 (Miwa Neishi actually repaired it with kintsugi, but that isn't visible in the photos); my great grandmother's silver sugar holder on page 89; my grandmother's forest plate on page 142 and cup on page 157; the cake server from my wedding on page 144; a pinch pot that I made on page 159; and teacups I made on page 74.

Friends and loved ones were also involved! My sister, Lauren Geyman, is the model on page 218, wearing earrings by Laura Lombardi; Ella Riley Adams is the model on page 160; and my daughter, Mona, is shown on page 159 with her crayon drawing and a custom couch cushion by Sarah Nsikak. The cushion is shown again on page 226. Loren Luzmore's mismatched teacups, from her friend Lois, come from West Germany and England, and are shown on pages 10, 96, 131, and 134.

I went to my parents' house in New Jersey the day before Fujio and I were set to photograph my grandmother's recipes. With my mom's help, I baked all of the recipes for that chapter, and with my dad's help, carefully packed them for safe transport to the shoot. Miraculously, it worked. Thank you to the many friends and family members who diligently recipe tested and made suggestions and comments.

Sometimes my daughter says, "I love everybody that I know." Parts of this project, and the team behind it, made me feel like that too! Thank you for being here.

Wishing you many, many sweet and peaceful tea times.

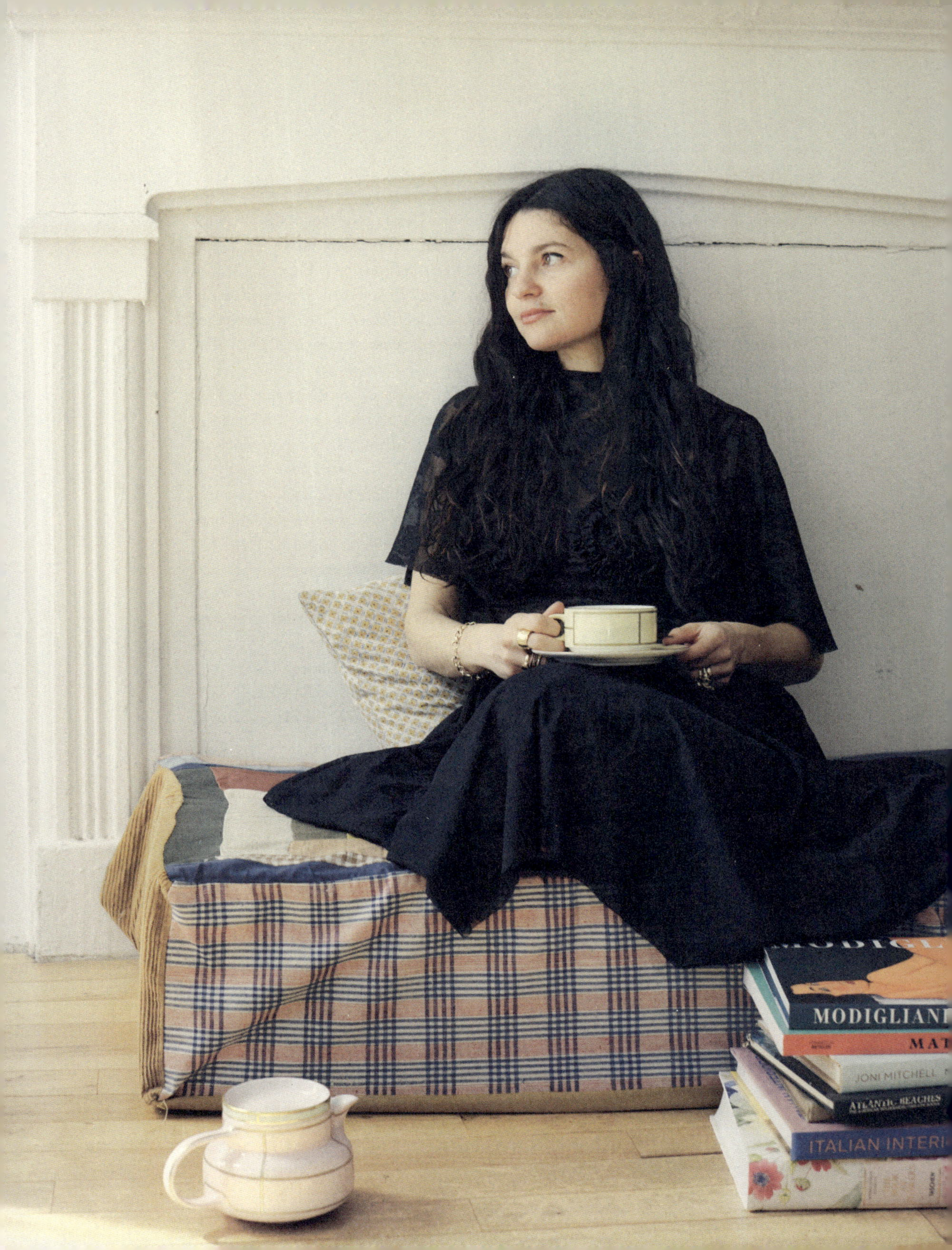
JONI MITCHELL
ATLANTIC BEACHES

About the Author

Maria Geyman is a board-certified naturopathic doctor and the founder of Masha Tea. She writes about travel, culture, fashion, and, of course, tea, with published work in *Vogue*, *Architectural Digest*, and *T Magazine*, as well as her newsletter *Tea for Two*. She occasionally consults for brands and hospitality groups on culture and wellness themes.

Born in Kiev, Ukraine, she grew up with the many tea sets that her family brought with them to New York during immigration. Her perspective comes from this lineage, from her summers picking flowers and berries in upstate New York, from travels to tea-growing parts of the world, and from graduate studies in Portland, Oregon, at the oldest naturopathic medical school in the country. Her perspective on tea culture is a vision for an international lifestyle that encompasses beauty, wellness, and strong relationships. *With Tea* is her first book.

She lives in Brooklyn, New York, with her wonderful husband, Ev, and her beautiful daughter, Mona.

First published in the United States of America in 2026 by
Rizzoli International Publications, Inc.
49 West 27th Street
New York, NY 10001
www.rizzoliusa.com

Watercolors: Alice Waese
Photography: Fujio Emura
Photographs by Maria Geyman pages 28, 37, 41, 42, 56, 59, 93, 222

Publisher: Charles Miers
Associate Publisher: James Muschett
Editor: Tricia Levi
Design: Jan Derevjanik
Production Manager: Colin Hough-Trapp
Managing Editor: Lynn Scrabis
Copyeditor: Sarah Scheffel
Proofreader: Sarah Stump

Cover: Kintsugi by Miwa Neishi

ISBN: 978-0-7893-4670-4
Library of Congress Control Number: 2026934553

Printed in China
2026 2027 2028 2029/ 10 9 8 7 6 5 4 3 2 1

The authorized representative in the EU for product safety and compliance is Mondadori Libri S.p.A., via Gian Battista Vico 42, Milan, Italy, 20123, www.mondadori.it

Visit us online:
Instagram: @RizzoliBooks
Facebook.com/RizzoliNewYork
Youtube.com/user/RizzoliNY